D1447933

The Diagnosis
and Treatment of
Epilepsy

The Diagnosis and Treatment of
Epilepsy

Richard Lechtenberg, M.D.
Associate Professor of Clinical Neurology
State University of New York
Downstate Medical School
Brooklyn, New York

MACMILLAN PUBLISHING COMPANY
NEW YORK

Collier Macmillan Canada, Inc.
TORONTO

Collier Macmillan Publishers
LONDON

Allen County Public Library
Ft. Wayne, Indiana

Copyright © 1985, Macmillan Publishing Company, a division of Macmillan, Inc.

Printed in the United States of America

All rights reserved. No part of this book may be reproduced or
transmitted in any form or by any means, electronic or mechanical,
including photocopying, recording, or any information storage and
retrieval system, without permission in writing from the Publisher.

Macmillan Publishing Company
866 Third Avenue, New York, New York 10022

Collier Macmillan Canada, Inc.
Collier Macmillan Publishers • London

Library of Congress Cataloging in Publication Data

Lechtenberg, Richard.
   The diagnosis and treatment of epilepsy.

   Includes bibliographical references and index.
   1. Epilepsy. I. Title. [DNLM: 1. Epilepsy—
diagnosis. 2. Epilepsy—therapy. WL 385 L4596d]
RC372.L37 1985   616.8'53   83-46180
ISBN 0-02-369080-1

Printing: 1 2 3 4 5 6 7 8   Year: 5 6 7 8 9 0 1 2 3

7137879

To Dr. Eli S. Goldensohn

Preface

This is a practical book written for the physician primarily responsible for the patient with seizures, whether that physician is a neurologist, family physician, gynecologist, pediatrician, general surgeon, or internist. Basic strategies for investigating and treating patients with epilepsy are discussed in an accessible but not oversimplified fashion for the benefit of the nonneurologist who does not see this kind of patient every day. The concepts underlying investigative techniques such as electroencephalography, computed tomography of the head, digital subtraction angiography, and positron emission tomography, as well as their limitations, are also discussed briefly, so that the physician who does not use these techniques regularly may gain some perspective on what can and should be done to study the individual with seizures.

Although any physician working in the area of seizure disorders knows that it often is difficult to extract a consensus from the range of views currently presented in the many publications on epilepsy, this book offers the most widely held views on diagnosis and treatment. It is a distillation of current thoughts and proven clinical approaches to seizure disorders.

Contents

The Diagnosis and Treatment of Epilepsy

1. Epilepsy: Facts and Fiction

Epilepsy usually can be managed successfully if it is diagnosed accurately, but both the diagnosis and treatment of epilepsy have been complicated by misconceptions that persistently surround this neurologic disorder. These misconceptions of epilepsy, its cause, management and prognosis, are held by both patients and physicians. This is not because epilepsy is rare. In fact, this neurologic disorder is relatively common and most physicians are obliged to diagnose, treat, or advise patients with recurrent seizures. The misconceptions surrounding this neurologic disorder probably persist because there is so much erroneous information, rather than simple ignorance, incited by fear of this very common problem. Nonphysicians have routinely viewed epilepsy as devastating and often intractable, and physicians have perceived the information on this disorder to be complex and usually inscrutable. Both of these views are inaccurate.

The physician principally responsible for the patient's general medical care is in the best position to dispel the patient's misconceptions and manage the patient's neurologic disorder. Usually the patient's primary physician, whether an internist, pediatrician, family practitioner, gynecologist, neurologist or other specialist, can most accurately assess the patient's complaints and treat the patient's problems on a long-term basis. Most seizure disorders can be managed easily and appropriately by physicians who are not epileptologists. Where a treatment plan follows accepted practice and fails to control an individual's seizures, the problem is as often with the patient's adherence to the physician's recommendations as it is with the physician's therapeutic approach.

Most seizure disorders can be well controlled with medication and attention to lifestyle. Unfortunately, it is the patient's misinformation and fears that often create the greatest barriers to effective treatment. Even when the physician primarily responsible for the person with epilepsy makes a reasonable diagnosis and provides the best available treatment for the affected individual, control of the epilepsy may be frustrated by the patient's incomplete or inconsistent cooperation. Complications develop in many cases years after the patient's initial evaluation and treatment. It is the nature of the disorder and the medications used to control it that make epilepsy a problem that cannot simply be treated and forgotten. Regular medical follow-up and continuing patient cooperation are essential in the management of epilepsy.

Epilepsy is a widespread medical problem. At least 1 of every 200 people in the United States and as many as 3 of every 200 in Europe have this neurologic disorder [1–3]. Although it often is viewed and treated as a single entity, epilepsy is actually a family of neurologic problems with overlapping characteristics. There is no one clinical trait that appears in all forms of epilepsy. The signs and symptoms exhibited during an episode of disturbed neurologic functioning and the changes in electrical activity detectable in the brain during that episode are what best define a neurologic problem as a type of epilepsy [4]. Recurrent episodes of inappropriate electrical activity in the brain, which interfere with central nervous system functioning, are presumed to be typical of every case of epilepsy. No pattern of behavior or movement is proof of seizure activity. Even patients with frequent seizures routinely exhibit no signs of neurologic disease between obvious attacks and may exhibit inconsistent deficits during seizures. This simply means that the diagnosis of epilepsy cannot be made confidently on the basis of clinical observations alone. Electrical studies are invaluable, but they too are not invariably conclusive.

Attempts to diagnose and manage epilepsy date back centuries, and consequently much of the confusion surrounding this disorder arises from the varied, and often archaic, terminology that has been used in discussions of epilepsy. There are some terms appropriately and many inappropriately equated with the term epilepsy. *Seizures* is not a synonym for epilepsy, even though seizures are the most basic feature of epilepsy. A depressed patient treated with electroconvulsive therapy has recurrent seizures, but does not have epilepsy by virtue of those induced seizures. However, because the episodes of disturbed brain function that underlie all types of epilepsy are called seizures, these neurologic disorders are also referred to as *seizure disorders*. Seizures often are loosely called *convulsions,* but a convulsion is a type of seizure in which prominent limb or trunk movements occur. Because common usage extended the meaning of this term to any type of epilepsy, drugs used to suppress epileptic attacks became known as *anticonvulsant medications.* These are more accurately called *antiepileptic drugs,* but the two names have become interchangeable. Although convulsion is a general term for several very different types of epileptic episodes, it is more descriptive and precise than colloquial references to seizures as *fits, drop attacks, blackout spells,* and *apoplexy.* These colloquialisms are used commonly by people without medical backgrounds and often confuse seizures with syncope. They are too imprecise to be used in any discussion of epilepsy. The same may be said of several terms used by neurologists and other physicians, but their familiarity has forced them into medical jargon. Some very old terms, such as *grand mal, petit mal,* and *absences,* are still widely used to describe seizures, even though they generally are not used in modern classifications of epilepsy without some descriptive qualifications. Because they are familiar to most physicians, these classic terms will be used along with currently accepted terminology throughout this book in the discussions of different types of epilepsy.

Along with a more consistent terminology for epilepsy has come a more widespread consensus on the criteria that must be met before a patient is given that diagnosis. Most physicians agree that one seizure does not establish the diagnosis of epilepsy. An individual must have more than one seizure or exhibit an unequivocal tendency to have seizures to be designated as having epilepsy. In special cases, such as seizures associated with high fevers in infants or recurrent electrical shocks in adults, even the appearance of more than one seizure during an individual's life does not establish the diagnosis of epilepsy. With few exceptions, epilepsy is a chronic disorder in which seizures recur if precautions or medications are not taken to prevent them. When a seizure does occur with no obvious provocation, the likelihood that that seizure will recur runs as high as 80 percent [1]. The diagnosis of epilepsy is reached only after careful evaluation of the patient and the patient's problem. The consequences of this diagnosis are far-reaching in both emotional and practical terms. Once the diagnosis is made, the patient is committed to treatment for years or for life [5]. If the diagnosis is publicized, the patient may face social and professional sanctions.

CLINICAL CHARACTERISTICS

What occurs during a seizure is distinctly different in each type of epilepsy. In some types of seizures, the patient will have no warning of an impending attack, will lose consciousness abruptly, and will develop violent jerking movements of the arms and legs. In others, the patient may exhibit nothing more than a blank stare or transient deviation of the eyes to one side. Some people experience hallucinations, unprovoked emotions, visual distortions, autonomic abnormalities, or compulsory behavior associated with their seizures. Still others have opisthotonic posturing, urinary or fecal incontinence, and forceful jaw contractions. All of these clinical characteristics occur in a variety of combinations in different people, but, for a particular individual, the pattern the seizure follows is likely to be fairly consistent. As the person with epilepsy matures, if he is a child, or ages, if he is an adult, the type of seizure that he displays may change dramatically. That an individual has one type of epilepsy does not bar or protect him from developing other types.

Epilepsy can be classified into broad categories according to the features of the seizures that consistently appear with each attack. Individuals with epileptic attacks that differ substantially from one episode to the next usually have mixed epilepsies—that is, a combination of distinct epilepsy types. Children with brief staring spells may also have generalized convulsions, in which case the child has a mixed seizure type, which most often proves to be a combination of generalized tonic-clonic (grand mal) and generalized absence (petit mal) epilepsy. Adults often have stereotyped behavior at the beginning of their seizures (complex partial epilepsy), with tonic-clonic movements at the end. The patient who always has only one type of seizure is certainly not rare, but most patients will experience two or more types of seizures during their lifetimes.

Many diagnoses are based on the signs and symptoms occurring during the seizure, but this information is not sufficient if the physician plans to treat the seizures. Even when the patient's attacks are distinctive, electrical studies of the brain are needed to determine the precise type of epilepsy responsible for the observed change in nervous system function. Accurate identification of the seizure type is vital in formulating a treatment plan. The type of epilepsy determines both the most likely prognosis and the most efficacious treatment.

Neurophysiologic Bases

Coordinated activity of nerve cells in the cerebral cortex is required for normal central nervous system function. When neuronal activity becomes disorganized, the physiologic disturbance usually will cause problems with consciousness, sensation, strength, or coordination. During a seizure or epileptic attack, brain function is upset by focal or generalized disturbances in neuronal activity. The type of impairment that occurs is determined by the location and severity of the nerve cell disturbance, which accounts for the remarkable variety of seizure disorders. The different forms that epilepsy may assume often have little more in common than that they all involve the disorganized or untimely discharge of many nerve cells in the cerebral cortex.

Seizure Threshold

What will provoke a seizure is as variable as the form the seizure activity may assume. Starvation, dehydration, and exhaustion may be required to precipitate seizures in one person, whereas flashing lights or one night of sleep deprivation may suffice in another patient. The point at which a seizure will occur is called the *seizure threshold*. This is a somewhat abstract concept, since all that can be said for a particular person with epilepsy is which stimuli will precipitate seizures most of the time. The person who experiences seizures after little provocation is said to have a low threshold. The threshold is unrelated to the type of epilepsy the individual has and may change as the patient ages. Everyone has a seizure threshold: For every person, there is a stimulus or combination of stimuli that will elicit seizures. People considered nonepileptic are those whose seizure thresholds are not reached by routine stresses and traumas.

Some structural and metabolic abnormalities in the brain will predictably lower seizure thresholds. A brain tumor, vascular malformation, or central nervous system infection will invariably increase a person's susceptibility to seizure activity. Hypocalcemia or hypoglycemia will induce seizures in most people if the serum level of calcium or glucose is dropped to an adequately provocative level.

Correcting electrolyte or glucose disorders will stop the accompanying seizures in most patients, but eliminating other types of acute problems, such as meningitis or intracranial bleeding, does not restore the patient's previous seizure threshold. In the patient with an acute meningitis, seizures may be provoked by little more than flashing lights when the infection is active, but even after the meningitis has been cured, the patient may have seizures provoked by 48 hours of sleep deprivation or relatively minor head trauma.

Most agents that lower the seizure threshold will be obvious from associated problems or neurologic signs that are present. A ruptured aneurysm will produce a subarachnoid hemorrhage that will lower the seizure threshold, but that hemorrhage also will produce changes in the patient's alertness or strength, as well as bloody cerebrospinal fluid. A brain tumor may produce seizures, but it also will usually produce weakness or psychological changes. Any individual with epilepsy who exhibits signs of persistent neurologic difficulty between seizure episodes must be investigated for a structural, infectious, or metabolic basis for the epilepsy.

Idiopathic and Symptomatic Seizures

All seizures are either idiopathic or symptomatic. Idiopathic seizures have no apparent basis, whereas symptomatic seizures are the manifestation of an identifiable problem. Most of the epilepsies that start at about the time of puberty are idiopathic. (Table 1–1). Those that develop in association with brain tumors, strokes, nervous system infections, head injuries, metabolic disorders, and congenital malformations of the brain are symptomatic. This distinction is important, because these two major groups have very different prognoses and require different therapies.

An individual with any of the common seizure types may have idiopathic or symptomatic seizures. That an individual has generalized tonic-clonic (grand mal) seizures does not exclude the possibility that the seizures are secondary

Table 1–1.
Seizure Categories

Idiopathic	Symptomatic
Normal brain structure	Evidence of head trauma, meningitis, metabolic disease, stroke, or the like
Normal neurologic examination	Dementia, paresis, sensory deficits, and so on are likely
Occasional familial pattern	Inheritance determined by associated disease
Typical age of onset	Appears within days or years of brain injury

to (i.e., symptomatic of) systemic lupus erythematosus. In contrast, the seizures of an individual with sarcoidosis or cysticercosis are not necessarily from central nervous system involvement with the sarcoid granulomas or the parasitic cysts. Patients with systemic problems that can cause seizures may have either idiopathic or symptomatic seizures. Management of the epilepsy or the systemic disease must take into account that the two problems *may be* related, but it cannot be based on the assumption that they *are* related.

In most cases, the prognosis with idiopathic seizures is better than that with symptomatic seizures. This simply means that when an obvious problem is causing epilepsy, it is more likely to complicate the management and course of the patient than when there is no apparent basis for the seizures. A patient whose seizures are caused by a brain tumor is not going to have as uneventful a course as the patient with idiopathic epilepsy. With both categories of epilepsy, the established explanation for the epilepsy must be recognized as nothing better than the best explanation to date, since what is presumed to be idiopathic may subsequently prove to be symptomatic.

The Variety of Seizure Disorders

Epilepsy has been divided and subdivided according to many different schemes. Terms familiar to most physicians and patients, such as *grand mal* and *petit mal,* have been replaced by names meant to indicate the physiologic basis for the seizure disorder. Whatever terminology is used to describe seizures must take into account the subtle varieties that constitute clinically similar disorders. The staring spells of petit mal or absence attacks occur with classic petit mal (see Chapter 2) as well with some types of *psychomotor* seizures. The generalized convulsions of grand mal epilepsy occur with many unrelated seizure disorders. The reports from people who observe the attacks can be misleading, especially if the observers have prejudices about what types of seizures can occur. Someone who equates staring spells with generalized absence (petit mal) seizures easily overlooks the postictal confusion in the patient who actually had a complex partial (psychomotor) seizure in which absence is a prominent feature.

Table 1–2.
Seizure Types

Proper Name	Common Name
Generalized	
Tonic-clonic[a]	Grand mal (major motor)
	Convulsive
Clonic[a]	
Tonic[a]	
Absence[b]	Petit mal
	Nonconvulsive
Impaired consciousness alone	
Mild clonic components	
Atonic components	
Tonic components	
Automatisms	
Autonomic signs	
Atypical absence[b]	Atypical petit mal
Pronounced changes in muscle tone	
Slow onset or cessation	
Atonic and akinetic[b]	Drop attacks
Myoclonic[b]	Impulsive petit mal
Partial	
Simple (elementary)	
Motor	Focal motor
Somatosensory or special sensory	Focal sensory
Autonomic	
Psychic	
Complex	Psychomotor
	Temporal lobe
With simple partial onset	
Impaired consciousness at start	
Secondarily generalized[a]	Sequential
Evolving from simple partial	
Evolving from complex partial	
Evolving from simple to complex partial	
Unclassified	

[a] Also called *convulsive seizures.*
[b] Also called *minor motor seizures.*

Most nonmedical people wrongly think of epilepsy as the convulsion of the generalized tonic-clonic seizure. In the convulsion, the patient has opisthotonic posturing, violent limb jerks, altered breathing, jaw clenching, and complete loss of consciousness. The suggestion that anything not involving these features is epilepsy is often greeted with skepticism by patients. This skepticism later is translated into poor compliance when medications with obvious side effects are prescribed for treatment of seizure disorders. The varieity of seizure disorders must be appreciated by any patient in whom epilepsy is diagnosed.

Although there is no internationally accepted scheme for naming epilepsies, there is one for naming seizures (Table 1–2) [4]. Currently, most neurologists studying or discussing epilepsy use the accepted name of the predominant seizure type observed to name the patient's epilepsy. Thus, people who usually have complex partial seizures are said to have *complex partial epilepsy*. However, this convention breaks down when several clearly different problems present with similar seizures. The simplest example of this is seizure activity in which prominent myoclonic limb jerks are the most obvious feature. Patients with either benign juvenile myoclonic epilepsy or photosensitive myoclonic epilepsy have myoclonic seizures, but the neurologic disorders have little else in common (see Chapter 2). Throughout this book, the internationally accepted terms for seizure types are used to refer to the various types of epilepsy, but it should be understood that many patients described as having one type of epilepsy experience more than one type of seizure.

COMMON MISCONCEPTIONS

The fears and fictions surrounding all types of epilepsy are innumerable [6]. None of these is new, but every misconception is a problem for the physician trying to develop a rational approach to the patient's disorder. Most cultures have traditionally viewed epilepsy as distinct from other chronic medical disorders, and this somewhat mystical conception of the disorder is still prevalent. Some cultures have ascribed epilepsy to divine intervention, some to satanic visitation, and others to humoral imbalances [6]. The reasons for its being accorded this special position are debatable: It may be because healthy individuals are struck down without warning or regard to their general health. Commonly held notions about individuals with epilepsy include that they are "mentally imbalanced, dull, or frankly mentally defective, liable to progressive mental deterioration, awkward to live with, antisocial or potentially criminal . . . " [7]. These notions are less pervasive than they were a few decades ago, but they still exist [8].

As a reaction to the distorted views about epilepsy that many people have, many physicians use euphemisms when discussing the disease with their patients. Patients are told that they have seizures, fits, attacks, or a seizure disorder, but not that they have epilepsy [6, 8]. Unfortunately, this simply compounds the problems. The ambiguous terms often confuse rather than comfort the person with epilepsy and reinforce the notion that epilepsy is too terrible to mention by name.

When an individual is told that he or she has epilepsy, an important part of that diagnosis must be an explanation of what epilepsy is and what problems the patient can expect as a consequence of the disorder. Many people believe that violent behavior is common in people with epilepsy, a misconception fostered by highly publicized court cases claiming an epileptic basis for antisocial or criminal behavior. The common notion that brain damage and epilepsy are inextricably linked must be addressed and dismissed. The risks of injury to the patient, the chances for control of the seizures, and the likelihood that the epilepsy will remit should all be discussed with the patient as soon as the diagnosis has been made.

INITIAL SIGNS

Often, diagnosing the specific type of epilepsy that an individual has is a bit complicated, but in some cases, simply making the diagnosis of epilepsy is difficult. Staring spells, peculiar movements, or involuntary posturing unassociated with a protracted or obvious loss of consciousness are routinely dismissed by friends and family of the patient as idiosyncrasies, tics, or nervousness. Obvious manifestations of seizure activity may be artfully concealed by the affected individual out of embarrassment or fear. Adults and children with seizures often have bed-wetting, nocturnal tongue biting, and transient losses of consciousness that lead to accidents months or years before they consult a physician. This response to the neurologic disorder is more from denial than deception. The affected person usually hopes that the problem will simply disappear.

Unfortunately, the consequences of denying this neurologic disorder may be tragic. If the seizures involve lapses in consciousness, the affected individual may be involved in a fatal automobile accident or crippling fall. Delays in diagnosis are especially common in very young and very old people. Old people with nocturnal incontinence often are thought to be senile, and children with staring spells often are dismissed as inattentive or mischievous. The elderly person who has a sudden loss of consciousness is mistakenly believed to have had a stroke, a development incorrectly viewed by many people as a reasonable consequence of senility. The child with more typical seizure activity usually receives medical attention.

CONCEALING EPILEPSY

Most people conceal the epilepsy from friends, family, and employers to avoid the sanctions that accompany this diagnosis [6]. If they admit to having epilepsy, most automatically lose their driver's licenses, at least temporarily, and they face substantial problems in securing many types of insurance [9]. Forty percent of people with epilepsy have difficulty getting a job, although almost 80 percent of the general population denies having any reservations about the employment of people with epilepsy [6, 8]. Even marriage becomes more of a problem because of the pressure exerted by families to discourage a family member's involvement with an epileptic individual [8].

Of course, much of the secrecy surrounding epilepsy originates with the patient's own prejudices. The more educated the patient, the less likely it is that he or she will allow the stigma associated with the disorder to be a real problem [10]. Because of this relationship between education and preoccupation with social stigma, children are especially vulnerable to feelings of shame associated with their condition. They often adopt a magical view of the seizure disorder, believing that it is their misbehavior which causes the epileptic attacks. Occasionally, these children are correct. The altered consciousness may entertain the children, and so they find ways to induce the seizures. Concealing these self-induced seizures may require considerable ingenuity, and this subterfuge reinforces the notion that something evil or unacceptable is instigating the seizures.

Patients with low seizure thresholds may risk having a seizure by purposely not taking their medication, if taking the medication provokes questions [11]. Young adults concerned about rejection by potential spouses may also hide their epilepsy. Still, the commonest setting in which people conceal epilepsy is at work. Patients least likely to complain of any stigma associated with their condition are those who have faced no employment discrimination or social limitations because of their disorder [10]. Although many patients worry about the consequences of telling their employer that they have epilepsy, only approximately 20 percent of those who do notify their employers experience any sanctions or special treatment [10]. Many of the reasons given by patients for taking extraordinary measures to conceal their epilepsy do not stand up to critical examination.

TREATMENT OPTIONS

Clearly, the patient's adjustment to epilepsy will be best if the seizures can be suppressed or eliminated. Epilepsy remits spontaneously in very few patients, but approximately 80 percent of patients will be completely or almost completely free of seizures with the use of antiepileptic medication. Since phenobarbital was introduced as a suppressant of seizure activity, the variety of effective antiepileptic drugs has been multiplying (see Chapter 14). For those patients who are incompletely controlled with medication or who tolerate the medication poorly, there are nonpharmaceutical approaches. These individuals may benefit from changes in lifestyle, surgery, dietary manipulation, biofeedback, or other techniques currently being developed, but no patient should be encouraged to believe that any of these are simpler or more effective than antiepileptic medications (see Chapter 15).

Antiepileptic drugs remain the first, and the best, option for controlling epilepsy. Despite the resistance of many patients to be dependent on a drug, alternative treatments do not have the proved success of these agents. Patients with epilepsy want a cure, not a palliative treatment. When patients refuse to take medication despite its established usefulness for them, it is usually because they want to shed all reminders of their neurologic disorder. The physician responsible for these patients must develop a strong alliance with them as part of the treatment plan, since every therapeutic regimen depends on patient compliance.

REFERENCES

1. Goodridge, D.M.G., Shorvon, S.D.   Epileptic seizures in a population of 6000. *Br. Med. J.* [Clin. Res.] 287:641–647, 1983.
2. Blumer, D.   Temporal lobe epilepsy and its psychiatric significance. In Benson, D.F., Blumer, D., (eds.), *Psychiatric Aspects of Neurologic Disease.* New York: Grune & Stratton, 1975, p. 171.
3. Berg, B.O.   Prognosis of childhood epilepsy—another look. *N. Engl. J. Med.* 306(14):861–862, 1982.
4. Commission on Classification and Terminology of the International League Against Epilepsy: Proposal for the revised clinical and electroencephalographic classification of epileptic seizures. *Epilepsia* 22:489–501, 1981.
5. Hauser, W.A., Anderson, V.E., Loewenson, R.B., et al.   Seizure recurrence after a first unprovoked seizure. *N. Engl. J. Med.* 307(9):522–528, 1982.
6. Burden, G.   Social aspects. In Reynolds, E.H., Trimble, M.R., (eds.), *Epilepsy and Psychiatry.* New York: Churchill Livingstone, 1981, pp. 296–305.
7. Fox, J.T.   The epileptic in industry. *Br. J. Phys. Med.* 11:140–144, 1948.
8. Caveness, W.F., Gallup, G.H., Jr.   A survey of public attitudes toward epilepsy in 1979 with an indication of trends over the past thirty years. *Epilepsia* 21:509–581, 1980.
9. Matthews, W.S., Barabas, G.   Suicide and epilepsy: a review of the literature. *Psychosomatics* 22(6):515–524, 1981.
10. Ryan, R., Kempner, K., Emlen, A.C.   The stigma of epilepsy as a self-concept. *Epilepsia* 21:433–444, 1980.
11. Lechtenberg, R.   *Epilepsy and The Family.* Cambridge, Mass.: Harvard University Press, 1984.

2. Types of Epilepsy

The pattern of epilepsy exhibited by any individual usually falls into one of several categories. Factors determining to which category the epilepsy belongs include the area of the brain that seems to be most involved by abnormal electrical activity, the sequence and assortment of signs and symptoms that occur during the seizure, and the progression of electrical changes in the brain that appear on the electroencephalogram during the episode. Some types of epilepsy occur only at specific ages, and so the age of the patient will also play a role in determining how these epilepsies are classified.

With some patients and some types of epilepsy, a full and accurate description of the symptoms and signs before, during, and after the typical seizure provides enough information to identify the type of epilepsy at least tentatively. The electroencephalogram will confirm or refute the clinical impression. Unfortunately, descriptions of these episodes usually are inaccurate and incomplete even when they are observed by physicians. This means that the physician is obliged to rely on the electroencephalogram. The electroencephalographic changes associated with a seizure are more objective than strictly clinical observations and can be recorded with fairly simple monitoring equipment. The major limitation of the electroencephalogram is that it is most informative when it includes samples of brain activity before, during, and after a seizure. The likelihood of obtaining this much information during a random observation lasting less than several hours is small, and in evaluating most patients with epilepsy, the usefulness of the information that *is* obtained may be negligible. As seizures become less frequent, documenting and analyzing them becomes more difficult.

Hence, the seizure classification, like any diagnosis, is subject to revision as more information about the episodes becomes available [1]. This in no way diminishes the importance of accurately classifying the seizures observed. Identifying the seizure type is the first step in deciding on treatment and anticipating problems. This is true whether the individual with epilepsy is a child or an adult. That two different patients have one clinical phenomenon in common during their seizures does not mean that they will profit from use of the same drugs or will experience the same complications in the course of their epilepsy. For example, the treatment of and inconvenience caused by complex partial seizures in adults are very different from those for generalized tonic-clonic seizures, even though altered consciousness is characteristic of both seizure types.

Three of 4 patients with seizures will have clinical episodes and electroencephalographic findings typical of a specific type of epilepsy (Table 2–1) [2]. The remaining patients will have seizure disorders that are fairly idiosyncratic, difficult to characterize by current criteria, or poorly defined by current diagnostic techniques. Patients with more than one type of seizure usually will have a predominant seizure type or a spectrum of seizure types that characterize the type of epilepsy. Thus, the child with absence (staring) spells, myoclonic jerks, and generalized tonic-clonic seizures does not have three types of epilepsy but one—benign juvenile myoclonic epilepsy—that typically causes different types of seizure episodes. Some patterns of epilepsy do change with age. Therefore, the newborn who exhibits frequent limb jerks as the manifestation of a neonatal seizure must be reassessed as the pattern of seizures

Table 2–1.
Prevalence of Seizure Types in the General Population

Seizure Type	Frequency (%)
Generalized	**37.7**
Primary	28.4
Tonic-clonic	11.3
Absence	9.9
Myoclonic	4.1
Other	3.1
Secondary	9.3
Lennox-Gastaut syndrome	5.1
West syndrome	1.3
Other	2.9
Partial	**62.3**
Simple	10.0
Complex	39.7
Secondarily generalized	12.6

changes over the course of months or years. As the type of epilepsy changes, so does the type of treatment appropriate for the patient.

The epilepsies that can be most easily defined and categorized are either partial or generalized (see Table 1–1) [3]. Partial seizures start in a relatively small area of the brain and remain limited to the area of cortex in which they arise, extend to only part of the cerebral cortex, or generalize to the entire cerebral cortex. Even when the partial seizure secondarily generalizes, the focal origin of the attack will usually be evident from the patient's signs and symptoms or his electroencephalographic recordings [4].

The generalized seizure seems to start in the entire cortex at the same time. Although the brain wave changes evident with any generalized seizure appear simultaneously over the entire cerebral cortex, the clinical signs of the seizure vary dramatically from one type of epilepsy to another. With generalized tonic-clonic epilepsy, the most obvious clinical manifestation of the seizure is a convulsion; with generalized absence epilepsy, a staring spell.

GENERALIZED EPILEPSIES

Generalized seizures occur in 20 to 40 percent of all patients with epilepsy and they occur at all ages [2, 5]. They are much more common in children than in adults: one-fourth of epileptic adults, as opposed to more than one-half of epileptic children, have generalized epilepsy [2]. Although the commonest types of generalized seizures are the tonic-clonic and absence forms, there are several less common forms that usually are seen in children and may involve relatively minor motor signs [2]. These are often called *minor motor seizures,* a name that is a bit misleading since the seizures are a major problem for the affected infant or child.

Most idiopathic generalized seizures appear at fairly specific ages [6]. Those appearing earliest are the generalized seizures of the newborn period, whereas those appearing latest are the benign myoclonic epilepsies that surface when the patient is approximately 15 years of age and the generalized tonic-clonic seizures that begin at about 16 years of age [6].

With most generalized seizures, the patient will lose consciousness for seconds or hours, a lapse sometimes more obvious to those around the patient than to the affected individual. If the seizures occur frequently, they may severely impair the affected child or adult. The child is especially impaired by frequent generalized seizures, because recurrent seizure activity of many types can interfere with normal intellectual development even without causing any structural damage to the brain.

Most idiopathic generalized epilepsies have some type of familial pattern, and most genetically determined seizure disorders occur as generalized epilepsies [5]. Obviously, patients with generalized epilepsies must inherit something that causes the seizures, even though they are classified as idiopathic. At autopsy, in many patients with these seizures, fine structural abnormalities are evident that are beyond the resolution of radiologic techniques that can be used while the patient is alive [7]. The commonest abnormalities found are microdysgeneses (microscopic developmental irregularities) [7]. Focal areas of nerve cells may be misaligned or primitively structured. What is surprising in these generalized disorders is that the dysgenesis can be localized to only a few areas of the cerebrum. These microdysgeneses probably are just the most obvious expressions of diffuse developmental defects in the brains of the affected individuals.

The terminology used to describe generalized seizures has become very confusing over the years, because distinctions have been made inconsistently between a variety of nonconvulsive seizures. Throughout this book, *generalized absence seizure* is a term reserved for seizures characterized by a three-per-second or, less often, a two-to four-per-second spike–and–slow wave pattern on the electroencephalogram of the affected individual (Fig. 2–1). There have been many reports of children with generalized seizures in which the typical electroencephalographic pattern of classic absence seizures is absent but the

Figure 2–1.
During a generalized absence attack that lasted 7 seconds, this child had 3-per-second spike–and–slow wave discharges that began (B) with an abrupt loss of consciousness and ended (E) with an equally abrupt return to normal consciousness. The interval between the vertical broken lines is 1 second.

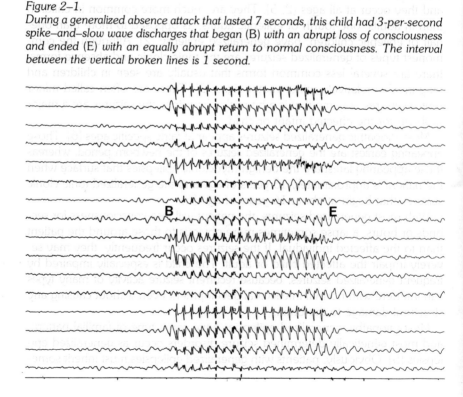

typical nonconvulsive attacks are present. These attacks are called *atypical absence* or *atypical petit mal* seizures to distinguish them from typical or classic absence seizures. The overabundance of similar terms has been further complicated by designating some types of partial seizures as *psychomotor absence.* In psychomotor absence attacks, the patient has clinical signs very much like those seen in the child or adult with generalized absence seizures, but the electroencephalographic pattern is that of a partial seizure and does not have the three per-second spike-and-wave or related pattern of the generalized (petit mal) absence attack.

These different terms have been used in the study of different groups of patients, and so any consideration of such groups makes their introduction unavoidable. For example, the mean age at onset of all types of absence seizures is approximately 4.3 years, but that for generalized (typical petit mal) absence seizures is approximately 7 years [6]. The atypical absence, rather than the psychomotor absence, seizures account for the earlier age at onset of all absence attacks.

Generalized Tonic-Clonic Epilepsy

Generalized tonic-clonic seizures (grand mal or convulsive seizures) appear in both children and adults as an abrupt loss of consciousness followed by convulsive movements of the body. They are usually idiopathic and often start in late childhood or adolescence [5]. Individual seizures may occur after an electrical shock or head injury, but most people with these seizures have recurrent episodes elicited by little or no obvious provocation. In other words, they have epilepsy.

This type of epilepsy has a good prognosis if the tonic-clonic seizures are the only type the patient exhibits. However, only 4 to 10 percent of patients with epilepsy have exclusively generalized tonic-clonic seizures [5].

The seizures themselves certainly are not rare, even though the strictly tonic-clonic epilepsy is somewhat uncommon. As many as 50 percent of patients with epilepsy have generalized tonic-clonic seizures at some time in their lives [5]. Individual seizure episodes usually are triggered by fatigue, sleep deprivation, or alcohol abuse in all except those with the lowest seizure thresholds [5]. Most of these individuals have other types of seizures that occasionally or routinely generalize. Although this epilepsy usually does not remit spontaneously, most patients (85 percent) with generalized tonic-clonic epilepsy alone are fully controlled with antiepileptic medications, such as phenytoin or valproic acid (see Chapter 13).

Clinical Features
The generalized seizures are called *tonic-clonic* or *clonic-tonic-clonic,* because there are two or three phases of muscle activity during the seizure proper or the *ictus* (Table 2–2).

17

Table 2–2.
Generalized Tonic-Clonic Seizures

Brief or no aura
Diffusely abnormal electroencephalogram initially and during ictus
Tonic posturing, clonic movements, or both
Tongue biting and other injuries common
Loss of consciousness
Cyanosis and altered breathing pattern
Bladder or bowel incontinence common
Ictus lasting 1 to 5 minutes
Postictal confusion usually lasting minutes

In the tonic phase, the patient has persistent or tonic contraction of several muscle groups; in the clonic phase, the contractions alternate repeatedly or clonically with abrupt relaxation. During the tonic phase, the patient usually arches his back and extends his arms and legs. Labored breathing or prolonged apnea and cyanosis during the first minute or two of the convulsion may foster concern that the airway is obstructed. Many patients who experience these seizures in a hospital are unnecessarily intubated at this point. The cyanosis and altered breathing pattern abate after a few minutes, although blood gases will still show a respiratory or metabolic acidosis that may persist for more than ½ hour after the tonic phase.

The seizure may begin with a massive jerk of the entire body or all the limbs, in which case it is more accurately described as clonic-tonic-clonic. In the tonic phase, the patient loses consciousness [5]. After this phase, more rhythmic jerking of the arms or legs or both may appear. These clonic movements may last seconds to minutes.

Injuries may occur for one of several reasons. Sometimes the patient inadvertently kicks solid objects that interfere with clonic limb movements. Some patients sustain injuries when they fall down at the beginning of the seizure. Older individuals with these episodes may develop spinal fractures from the force of the paraspinal muscle contractions. Patients of any age may suffer a shoulder dislocation or other joint injury from the abnormal contraction of muscles during either the clonic or the tonic phase of the seizure. Also, many individuals bite their tongue or lacerate their gums during the tonic phase. Nonetheless, most people with this type of generalized seizure do not injure themselves, although many have urinary incontinence and a few have fecal incontinence.

Electroencephalographic Features
When the seizure begins, the electrical pattern detected by electroencephalography over the entire cortex becomes simultaneously abnormal. Spikes and slow waves, often of very high amplitudes, develop synchronously in

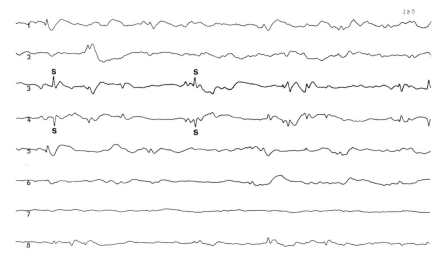

Figure 2–2.
Distinct spikes (s) *arose from several different areas of the cortex in this severely retarded child. These were obvious even when the child's generalized tonic-clonic seizures were well controlled.*

widely scattered areas of the cerebrum (see Chapter 6). The abnormal electrical activity in the brain, which is responsible for the seizure, and the metabolic changes associated with it do not cause brain damage, at least in older children and adults. The risk to the very young child is less well defined. Although most, if not all, patients with this type of seizure recover fully after an episode, the electroencephalographic abnormalities may persist after the patient has recovered consciousness, and some abnormalities often appear on recordings taken several hours or even days after the ictus (Fig. 2–2).

Postictal Period
The ictus in generalized tonic-clonic seizures lasts several seconds to a few minutes. Subsequently, the patient will be poorly responsive to all stimuli for minutes or hours, an interval called the *postictal period.* If seizures occur during sleep, a common setting for many different types of seizures, the individual may sleep through the postictal period. A person who experiences these seizures only when he is asleep may awake in the morning wondering why his tongue is sore or why there is urine in the bed. Many patients with nocturnal seizures complain of headaches in the morning and may find that they have a twisted ankle or unexplained bruises. When nocturnal bed-wetting (enuresis) occurs in children at about the time of puberty, it is often mistakenly ascribed to a transient regression rather than to a nocturnal seizure.

Generalized Absence Epilepsy

Generalized absence epilepsy (typical petit mal or nonconvulsive epilepsy) invariably appears first in childhood, usually in individuals between 6 and 12 years of age [8]. The principal feature of the disorder is a momentary loss of consciousness, which is called an *absence attack* [8]. This type of seizure occurs as the sole type of seizure exhibited by the affected individual in only 3 to 4 percent of all individuals who have epilepsy [5]. This statistic suggests that generalized absence epilepsy is fairly uncommon, which is certainly not true if children alone are considered. Generalized absence epilepsy changes as the child ages, and the child develops another type of seizure disorder or stops having seizures when he reaches adulthood [5, 9]. Fourteen percent of children with generalized absence seizures will also have generalized tonic-clonic seizures from the onset of the disorder [5]. Of those who have strictly absence seizures initially, 32 percent will develop tonic-clonic seizures later in life [5]. There is a strong familial pattern with this type of epilepsy, but some neurologists believe this is a group of similar seizure disorders, only some of which are hereditary [5].

Clinical Features
With classic absence attacks, the child has no warning of an impending seizure and usually is unaware that one has occurred (Table 2–3).

The typical episode involves little more than a staring spell during which the child is completely out of touch with the environment. If the child is speaking when a seizure occurs, he will simply become mute for the duration of the attack. Attacks rarely last more than 20 seconds. There is no loss of postural tone, and so the patient does not fall during the seizure. Eighty-eight percent of patients have some form of incidental movement, such as blinking, facial twitches, or chewing movements, during at least one attack [5]. The affected child is unaware that he has had a lapse in consciousness, even if he was involved in an activity requiring continuous attention. Because of the character of the seizures, absence attacks often occur for months or years before they are recognized as anything more than peculiar behavior.

Table 2–3.
Generalized Absence Seizures

No aura
Typical three-per-second spike–and–slow wave pattern on electroencephalogram
Maintained posture
Loss of consciousness
No incontinence
Subtle or no facial and limb movements
Ictus usually lasting 5 to 90 seconds
No postictal confusion

Electroencephalographic Features

Children with classic generalized absence seizures usually have a typical 3-Hz spike–and–slow wave pattern on the electroencephalogram during the seizures (see Fig. 2–1). This characteristic pattern also is seen often between actual seizures and may be induced by flashing lights or hyperventilation in susceptible individuals [8, 10, 11]. Less common patterns with otherwise typical attacks include 2- to 4-Hz spike–and–slow wave or polyspike-and-wave patterns (Fig. 2–3). These electroencephalographic patterns often appear when seizures are not occurring and may be found in relatives of the patient who never have seizures.

Postictal Period

There is no postictal period in true generalized absence seizures, a trait which helps distinguish this type of generalized seizure from certain types of partial seizures that can also cause staring spells with little more than chewing movements [5]. For example, complex partial seizures often are misdiagnosed as petit mal when they appear as episodes of confusion and aphonia in young adults [1] (see Table 2–3).

Even though the altered consciousness in generalized absence is transient, the frequency of the attacks may be substantial enough to interfere with learning. If the attacks occur several times per week or even several times per day, the child's intellectual development may be stunted. Despite this impaired development, patients who have normal intelligence quotient (I.Q.) scores early in childhood will have consistently normal scores even if the epilepsy persists for a decade [12]. That intellectual ability is preserved does not mean that intellectual development will not be impaired by recurrent seizures.

Other Generalized Epilepsies

Most other classifiable types of generalized seizures rarely occur after childhood (Table 2–4). Many of these are epilepsies that develop secondary to perinatal

Table 2–4.
Prevalence of Seizure Types in Patients Before and After 15 Years of Age

Seizure Type	Patients 0–15 Years Old (%)	Patients 15 Years Old or Older (%)
Generalized	**55.0**	**22.3**
Tonic-clonic	10.4	12.0
Absence	17.8	2.8
Myoclonic	3.7	4.4
Other	23.1	3.1
Partial	**45.0**	**77.7**
Simple	7.4	12.3
Complex	21.4	55.9
Other	16.2	9.5

or intrauterine brain damage from infection, ischemia, malformation, or hemorrhage. These are symptomatic epilepsies rather than idiopathic or primary. Some of the unusual forms of generalized seizures appearing in infancy or childhood are primary—that is, idiopathic—and follow familial patterns. Some types of generalized seizures routinely appear in association with other neurologic signs as part of syndromes. The most common of these are the West syndrome and the Lennox-Gastaut syndrome [2, 5].

West Syndrome

Infants with diffusely abnormal electroencephalograms, myoclonic jerks, frequent convulsions, and psychomotor retardation are said to have *West syndrome* [5, 13]. This is not truly a specific type of epilepsy but a disorder of which several kinds of peculiar generalized seizures are one facet [14]. The types of seizures that the affected infants exhibit are very different from the generalized seizures that appear later in childhood or adulthood. These seizures often involve paroxysms of jerking limb movements called *infantile spasms* (see Chapter 5). The types of seizures associated with infantile spasms all appear to be generalized.

The electroencephalogram typically seen in affected infants shows high-voltage spikes and waves arising from all parts of the cerebral cortex. The abnormal brain waves persist between apparent spasms and produce a characteristically disorganized electroencephalographic pattern called *hypsarrhythmia*. Infantile spasms with hypsarrhythmia are caused by several different types of neurologic disease, but they most often appear after perinatal trauma or asphyxia [13, 14]. West syndrome appears between 1 month and 3 years of age, but most infants exhibit their first infantile spasms at 3 to 7 months [2, 9, 14, 15]. Many of the children with this problem die, and most who survive are severely retarded [15].

Lennox-Gastaut Syndrome

With the Lennox-Gastaut syndrome, generalized seizures appear in children between 1 and 7 years old in association with myoclonic jerks and mental retardation [5]. As in the West syndrome, these are usually symptomatic seizures, and in some children, the Lennox-Gastaut syndrome may be a late variant of the West syndrome [2, 5]. These two syndromes are clearly not the same, but they do share some characteristics. The Lennox-Gastaut syndrome more often than not develops in children who have not had West syndrome and appears at a later age than is typical of the West syndrome [14]. It is resistant to treatment and has a variable association with retardation [14]. As in the West syndrome, causes of the Lennox-Gastaut syndrome include perinatal ischemia, hypoxia, intracranial hemorrhage, cytomegalovirus or toxoplasmosis infection, tuberous sclerosis, and many of the other causes of childhood epilepsy discussed in Chapter 5 [5].

Minor Motor Seizures

Infants may have generalized seizures in which body tone transiently disappears or peculiar postures briefly appear. These are called *minor motor seizures* (see Table 1–2) and range from akinetic attacks, in which the child exhibits no movements, to salaam attacks, in which the infant thrusts its arms forward and drops its head onto its chest. Some physicians consider the infantile spasms of West syndrome to be a form of minor motor seizure [15]. Minor motor seizures usually develop in the newborn period and invariably appear during the first few years of life. These seizures may progress to more complex forms as the child matures.

Myoclonic Seizures

There are many different types of generalized seizures with prominent myoclonus. Some of these are clearly hereditary and others exhibit no familial patterns. Although this is not a rare type of epilepsy, the variety of forms assumed makes it difficult to characterize as a group.

The most common type is benign juvenile myoclonic epilepsy. This is an idiopathic seizure disorder that usually appears at approximately 15 years of age [6]. It affects about 4 percent of all people with epilepsy, but it usually is not diagnosed until many years after it develops [6]. This delay of 8 to 9 years between onset and diagnosis is explained by the unusual pattern of the seizures. They begin as myoclonic jerks, primarily in the arms and only on awakening in the morning or after a nap (Table 2–5). As the disorder progresses, the myoclonic jerks become more frequent and appear during the day. They may be more frequent when the affected individual is tired, but they do not occur as he is falling asleep [6]. Consciousness is not impaired, except in the most severe episodes, and even then the impairment is fleeting. If they are standing, many people with this type of epilepsy fall when the myoclonic jerks occur. Photic stimuli and, much more rarely, auditory stimuli may trigger attacks.

As many as 40 percent of patients with benign juvenile myoclonic epilepsy will experience at least one episode of myoclonic status epilepticus, in which the attacks occur every few seconds and continue for minutes to hours [6]. This and more transient attacks of myoclonic seizures usually are precipitated

Table 2–5.
Benign Juvenile Myoclonic Epilepsy

No aura
Myoclonic jerks on awakening
High sensitivity to sleep deprivation
Often triggered by photic stimulation
No impairment of consciousness
No postictal confusion

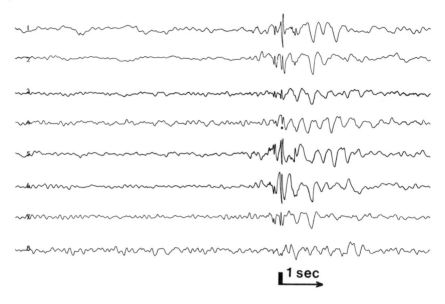

Figure 2–3.
This child with refractory seizures had recurrent generalized polyspike discharges of the sort occasionally seen with absence attacks.

by sleep deprivation. This type of status epilepticus is not associated with impaired consciousness [6].

Only 17 percent of patients with benign juvenile myolconic epilepsy have strictly myoclonic seizures [6]. Fifty-eight percent have generalized tonic-clonic seizures as well as myoclonus, and 25 percent have absence attacks, generalized tonic-clonic seizures, and myoclonus [6]. These absence attacks are probably atypical petit mal—that is, generalized nonconvulsive seizures with an irregular spike-and-wave pattern on the electroencephalogram and more pronounced changes in tone during the absence than is typical of classic absence attacks. The patient may also have a more protracted recovery from the seizure and a more abrupt onset of the episode than is typical for generalized absence attacks [3].

Approximately one-third of the patients with this disorder have abnormal brain wave activity elicited by photic stimulation [6]. During attacks and during photic stimulation, the electroencephalogram usually displays a generalized, paroxysmal, symmetrical polyspike–and–slow wave discharge (see Fig. 2–3).

Most patients with this type of epilepsy have a normal intellect and normal neurologic examinations [6]. Some investigators have found an increased incidence of personality disorders in patients with benign juvenile myoclonic epilepsy, but this is controversial [16]. The severity of the disorder abates as patients enter adult life, but it does not disappear completely. Even with complete seizure control by medication, there is considerable evidence that the epilepsy will recur within months or years of stopping the medication in most individuals [6].

PARTIAL EPILEPSIES

Most epilepsies that occur in adults are partial epilepsies. Approximately 62 percent of all patients with epilepsy and 78 percent of patients older than 15 years have partial epilepsies (see Table 2–4) [2]. These are often symptomatic but may be idiopathic. Many children with generalized seizures, especially those with generalized absence seizures, develop partial seizures during or after adolescence.

In all partial seizures, abnormal electrical activity starts in a limited area of the brain, most often, if not always, in the cerebral cortex. Partial seizures are

Figure 2–4.
Complex partial seizures often originate in the temporal lobe, but they may develop with lesions above the sylvian fissure (arrows) or elsewhere in the brain. This is a lateral view of a normal brain, with lobes and other landmarks indicated. (A. = artery.)

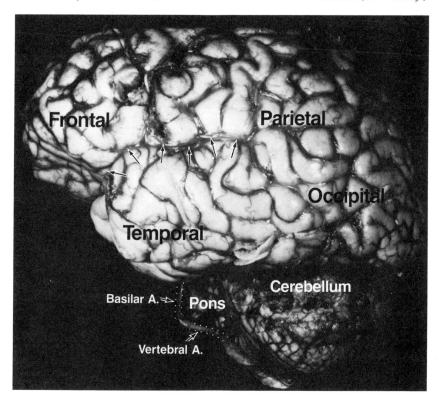

classified as simple or complex, depending on whether the seizure remains as a focal discharge and causes only motor, sensory, or autonomic signs, or the focal discharge spreads substantially and causes combinations of autonomic, motor, and sensory symptoms or altered or impaired consciousness [3]. If the partial seizure progresses to a generalized tonic-clonic seizure, it is said to be a simple or complex partial seizure that secondarily generalizes [17]. A seizure that begins in a small area of the cortex and spreads to virtually all of the cerebral cortex in less than a few seconds will resemble a primary, as opposed to a secondary, generalized seizure. These progressive seizures are also called *sequential seizures* because of the spread of abnormal electrical activity on the electroencephalogram obtained during the seizure [11].

Simple (or elementary) *motor* and *simple sensory seizures* are partial seizures with strictly motor or strictly sensory signs and symptoms. These have traditionally been called *focal motor* and *focal sensory* seizures. Lesions responsible for these simple motor or sensory seizures are likely to be in the occipital, parietal, or frontal cortex in areas devoted to relatively simple functions, such as perception of light or movement of a limb. Partial seizures in which complex autonomic, psychological, sensory, or motor signs and symptoms develop during the attacks are called *complex* partial seizures. These are better known as *psychomotor* or *temporal lobe* seizures. Most lesions producing complex partial seizures are in the temporal lobe (Fig. 2–4). Even when there is no obvious structural problem responsible for the seizures, the focus of epileptic activity defined by electroencephalographic studies is usually in the temporal lobe [18, 19].

Complex Partial Epilepsy

Partial seizures with complex symptomatology occur in both children and adults and are the most common type of partial seizure. Twenty to 30 percent of all people suffering from epilepsy have this form of partial seizure alone or in combination with other types of seizures [19]. Most of those who develop complex partial epilepsy have their first seizure at about the time of puberty [19]. These may be idiopathic or symptomatic, but if the seizures appear after adolescence, they generally are symptomatic of a structural brain lesion [17]. Up to 15 percent of all partial epilepsies appearing in patients between 30 and 60 years of age are from primary or metastatic brain tumors alone [17].

Temporal lobe epilepsy is a widely used but misleading name for this type of epilepsy. Seizures arising in the temporal lobe do not necessarily produce psychomotor seizures, and psychomotor seizures do not necessarily occur only with temporal lobe damage [11]. In fact, 20 to 25 percent of all complex partial seizure disorders seem to originate outside the temporal lobes [20]. In most patients with complex partial epilepsy, there is no apparent structural basis for the seizures [19].

Complex partial seizures may go unrecognized for years, because the signs

Table 2–6.
Complex Partial Seizures

Extremely diverse and often complex auras
Abnormality beginning focally on electroencephalogram
Possible loss of posture or abnormal limb movements
Possible altered or complete loss of consciousness
Possible prominent affective or cognitive disorder
Ictus lasting seconds to several minutes
Possible generalization to convulsive seizure
Postictal confusion lasting minutes to hours

and symptoms associated with these epileptic attacks are very diverse (Table 2–6). One-third of the patients who develop complex partial epilepsy exhibit these types of seizures only after having a generalized tonic-clonic, absence, or myoclonic seizure disorder for years [19]. Sixty-four percent of people with complex partial seizures have secondary or associated primary generalized seizures as well [19].

Every complex partial seizure has several discrete stages. As in generalized seizures, the stage with the most electrical disorganization apparent on the electroencephalogram is the ictus. This is often preceded by premonitory signs and symptoms, called the *aura*. The postictal period is similar to that exhibited by patients with generalized tonic-clonic seizures. The interval between obvious seizure activity is the interictal period.

The Aura

The character of the aura experienced by the patient often provides information on where the seizure is originating. These premonitory sensations or behavior are actually part of the seizure, but they are distinct from the ictus because of the way the patient perceives them. Usually, the seizure victim will remember the aura, even if everything transpiring during the ictus and the postictal period is forgotten. The aura will be perceived as a reliable indicator that a seizure is about to occur [21, 22]. Auras occur with other partial and some generalized seizures, but they are most common and most complex in complex partial seizures.

In some cases, the aura entails stereotyped behavior, (Table 2–7). The

Table 2–7.
Auras with Complex Partial Epilepsy

Gastrointestinal distress
Urgent need to defecate
Olfactory, auditory, or visual hallucinations
Intense fear
Automatisms involving face, limbs, or entire body
Feelings of depersonalization
Déjà vu or *jamais vu*

individual abruptly feels compelled to make some type of movement or perform some familiar act. He must turn his head, lift his arm, or sit down. Sometimes, the affected individual will demand, pour, or drink water [23]. Chewing movements, lip smacking, spitting, or grimacing may all occur as part of the aura [21].

The altered behavior or perceptions of the aura may not be distinctly different from those experienced during the ictus, but the signs and symptoms in both of these periods will loosely relate to the area of the brain that seems to have the most abnormal electrical activity at the time. When the focus of the seizure is in the frontal lobe, especially in the area overlying the orbits, the patient may complain of olfactory hallucinations, excessive sweating, a rapid pulse, or increased gastrointestinal motility [17]. With foci more clearly in the temporal lobe, the patient will report visual delusions, such as micropsia or macropsia, altered time sense, altered depth perception, or vertigo [17, 24, 25].

Sometimes the aura seems to originate in specific temporal lobe systems, such as that including the uncus, amygdala, and hippocampus, in which case the seizures are called *uncinate seizures*. With this uncinate form of complex partial seizures, the patient complains of a disagreeable smell or taste [21]. Complaints of nausea or abdominal cramps are also fairly common in uncinate attacks. These uncinate auras have slightly more significance than other auras, because with them, the likelihood of an unsuspected tumor in the temporal lobe of the brain is increased [23].

Psychological complaints are common with seizures originating in the temporal lobe and include feelings of detachment and unreality [20]. Auditory hallucinations occur in some auras. The patient usually hears music or a buzzing sound, but occasionally, the noises are more menacing and involve threatening voices. Visual hallucinations occur less often than auditory hallucinations [26, 27]. Some patients complain of paranoid ideas, persecutory delusions, and ideas of reference [24, 28]

More characteristic of complex partial auras are the feelings of intense familiarity with events just occurring or total unfamiliarity with events that have occurred many times before [19]. These are called déjà vu and *jamais vu*, respectively, and often occur in people who exhibit no neurologic or psychiatric problems. What makes them significant in individuals with complex partial seizures is that they appear repeatedly just before a seizure occurs.

Other phenomena occurring during the aura that are more clearly abnormal include embarrassing automatic activities, such as undressing or urinating [26]. Attacks of intense groundless fear sometimes also occur during the aura [29].

The Ictus
The ictus in complex partial epilepsy may be just a prolonged staring spell or it may generalize to a tonic-clonic seizure. The seizure will always involve more than just a staring spell if it originates in areas outside the temporal

lobes [20]. Fairly complex but purposeless behavior such as undressing, running, laughing, or crying may occur [19, 27, 30]. Some patients have sexual climax during the seizure, but this is extremely rare and usually seen only in patients whose seizures are triggered by sexual excitement [19].

During the ictus, the patient may not fully lose consciousness, but he invariably has profoundly altered consciousness. He should remember little or none of the ictus when he recovers. The ictus of a complex partial seizure lasts seconds to minutes and usually is not associated with incontinence unless the seizure secondarily generalizes. During the ictus, the patient usually makes purposeless movements but occasionally also wanders aimlessly, speaks in unintelligible phrases, drinks water, urinates, defecates, or simply hides [23]. If the seizure generalizes, the patient may bite his tongue, experience urinary incontinence, and exhibit clonic muscle activity.

The Postictal Period
The postictal period is the interval between the ictus and the return to normal consciousness. It lasts 2 to 10 minutes in most complex partial seizures and is characterized by disorientation and inattention but very little activity [22, 28, 31]. Some patients will be unaware that any alteration in consciousness occurred, if the ictus and postictal period are fairly brief [19]. If the seizure generalizes, the patient will realize that something abnormal has occurred and may exhibit a great deal of irritability during the postictal period.

Violent or aggressive behavior during this period is fairly uncommon, but some patients do injure themselves or damage property while in this confused state [19, 32]. If the patient exhibits destructive behavior, he will usually not remember the violence. Confused but nonviolent behavior that occasionally occurs during the postictal period includes undressing and sexually provocative acts. Such behavior is easily recognized as purposeless [19].

The Interictal Period
The interval that does not include the aura, ictus, or postictal period of the seizure is called the *interictal period*. During this interval, the patient is, by definition, free of all seizure activity. There is still controversy regarding whether long-term effects of the epilepsy, especially with complex partial epilepsy, are apparent during this seizure-free interval [18, 33]. Some physicians believe that new personality traits and psychological problems may appear during the interictal period of complex partial seizures after the patient has had complex partial epilepsy for years or decades [24, 34, 35].

Simple Partial Epilepsy

Simple partial seizures are partial seizures with focal motor, sensory, or autonomic signs and symptoms. These seizures may produce few signs typically associated with epilepsy and may appear as nothing more than a focal sensory change or an abnormal limb movement. If the abnormality is always so limited with each attack, the patient has simple partial motor (focal motor) or sensory (focal sensory) epilepsy. During these simple partial seizures, the patient usually remains alert, even if part of a limb or an entire limb has rhythmic involuntary contractions. In one type of partial epilepsy, the abnormal motor or sensory activity starts in a very limited area and becomes generalized [10]. For example, twitching in the thumb may spread to the arm and lead to a generalized tonic-clonic convulsion in a jacksonian "march" or jacksonian seizure [11, 36]. The seizure disorder is considered a simple or elementary partial seizure even if the initially focal movement spreads or generalizes [15].

Simple partial seizures are very different from complex partial seizures in their course, complications, and clinical signs. There is clearly no increased incidence of psychological disturbances with focal motor, focal sensory, and jacksonian seizures [37]. Spontaneous remission is the rule with some types of simple partial epilepsy.

Rolandic Epilepsy

In one form of focal epilepsy called *benign focal epilepsy of childhood* or *rolandic epilepsy,* the seizure disorder remits by the end of adolescence. This is a fairly common childhood epilepsy, accounting for 15 percent of all child-hood seizure disorders [5]. It usually presents with a nocturnal seizure that starts with focal motor signs but involves tonic-clonic movements. These nocturnal seizures first appear in children 5 to 9 years of age. As these children mature, seizures occur while they are awake, and often there is hemifacial twitching or clonic movements in one arm initially [5]. Oropharyngeal involvement may appear as a speech arrest at the start of the seizure.

The electroencephalographic changes with rolandic epilepsy are fairly consistent. The interictal record shows high-voltage spikes followed by slow waves, singly or in groups, clustered about the rolandic fissure (Fig. 2–5) [5]. The rolandic fissure separates the frontal lobe from the parietal lobe.

This type of epilepsy is inherited in an autosomal dominant pattern [5]. That penetrance is variable is evident from the high incidence of abnormal electroencephalographic patterns in siblings; 34 percent of an affected individual's brothers and sisters will have rolandic spikes, even if they never have seizures [5]. Even before remission, this type of epilepsy is easily suppressed with drugs [8].

COMBINATIONS OF SEIZURE TYPES

Two or more patterns of seizures often occur in people with epilepsy. Certain types of seizures are associated with one another more often than others. The most common combination will involve partial seizures that secondarily

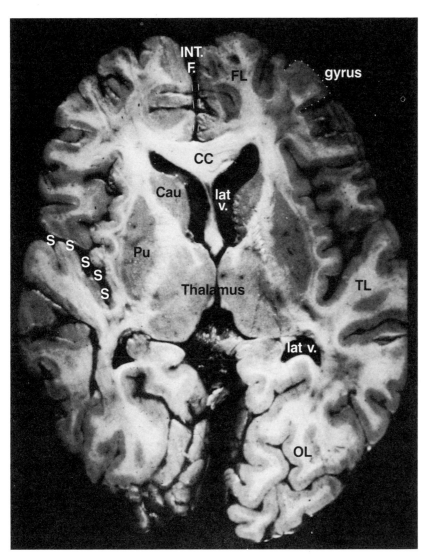

Figure 2–5.
This horizontal section of the brain reveals the anterior portion of the interhemispheric fissure (INT. F.), which extends between the cerebral hemispheres to the corpus callosum (CC). The sylvian fissure (S) separates the temporal lobe from the island of Reil. Additional landmarks include the lateral ventricle (lat v.), the thalamus (right and left), the head of the caudate nucleus (Cau), and the putamen (Pu). The frontal (FL), temporal (TL), and occipital (OL) lobes are cut in the plane of the section.

generalize. In most patients with the jacksonian march phenomenon, a generalized tonic-clonic seizure will evolve as part of the episode. Complex partial seizures often progress to generalized tonic-clonic seizures. The child with generalized nonconvulsive epilepsy may experience episodes of complex partial seizures as he or she matures. For any patient with more than one seizure type, the treatment must be tailored to the particular seizure types that are most apparent (see Chapter 13).

SEIZURES WITH MENSTRUATION

Seizures occurring during the luteal phase of the menstrual cycle are not a distinct type of epilepsy, although they are routinely called *catamenial seizures* [38]. Women may develop these seizures at the same time every month as a result of hormonal changes. Presumably, the seizure threshold falls cyclically along with other changes induced by the menstrual cycle. Water retention, electrolyte changes, and falling progesterone levels all help trigger catamenial seizures [38]. These seizures often are generalized, but different seizure types have been associated with the period of menstrual flow. Based on the assumption that low levels of progesterone contribute to the lowered seizure thresholds, many women have been given supplemental progesterone when they most often develop seizures, but the effect of this approach on seizure frequency has not been obvious [38]. In managing this type of epilepsy, it is best to make cyclic adjustments in the antiepileptic drugs used (see Chapter 13).

STATUS EPILEPTICUS

If seizures occur repeatedly so that the patient does not return to his usual level of functioning between episodes, the condition is called *status epilepticus*. The most common seizure type that occurs as status epilepticus is the generalized tonic-clonic seizure. With this disorder, the patient usually is unresponsive between obvious tonic-clonic episodes. There are types of status epilepticus, such as absence or complex partial status epilepticus, in which the patient responds, albeit in a confused or inappropriate manner, during the episode; and there are other types in which consciousness is minimally impaired. That status epilepticus is the problem in any of these situations is suggested by clinical signs of recurrent or persistent seizure activity, which can be corroborated by electroencephalographic studies whenever the basis for the patient's altered behavior or consciousness is unclear.

The clinical signs exhibited by the patient may change during status epilepticus, even if the type of electrical disturbance in the brain remains constant. The patient with generalized tonic-clonic status epilepticus that persists for several hours or days may have progressively less movement associated with each discrete attack. Tonic deviation of the eyes to one side or a paroxysm of nystagmus and facial twitching may be the only evidence of the seizures. This probably represents a variety of transformations occurring in the brain as the entire system fatigues from the constant strain of inappropriate electrical activity.

The types of status epilepticus in which the patient suffers little apparent impairment of consciousness even while intractable seizure activity occurs are less common than the types in which the patient is in coma for the duration of the episode. Nonetheless, there are several forms of epilepsy that can cause status epilepticus with persistent consciousness. One fairly common form in which the patient is alert and responsive is myoclonic status epilepticus, a complication of benign juvenile myoclonic epilepsy [6]. With status epilepticus secondary to simple partial motor seizures also, the patient is awake, even if the seizures interfere with purposeful activity. Clarity of thinking may be impaired with the simple partial motor seizures, even though consciousness appears to be fairly normal. If the simple partial seizures last for days, the episode often is called *epilepsia partialis continua,* a very old name that remains in common use.

Complex partial and generalized absence seizures very rarely appear as status epilepticus, but when they do, the diagnosis may be impossible to make without obtaining an electroencephalogram [39, 40]. Status epilepticus with these types of epilepsy usually is manifest as confusion, aphasia, automatisms, and other fairly nonspecific signs and symptoms that suggest psychosis more than neurologic disease [39, 41]. These are called *nonconvulsive status epilepticus,* because the tonic-clonic activity so typical of status epilepticus with generalized convulsions is absent [39].

During both complex partial and generalized absence (petit mal or nonconvulsive) status epilepticus, the electroencephalogram will reveal ongoing or recurrent seizure activity [29, 40]. This is diagnosed as status epilepticus, rather than just a prolonged seizure, if the abnormal activity persists for more than 30 minutes without ever returning to the baseline functioning evident before the episode began [39]. Whereas the long-term effects of complex partial status epilepticus are unknown, there is evidence that generalized absence status epilepticus in early childhood may cause brain damage [42]. That the status epilepticus is not a convulsive disorder does not mean it is benign.

Generalized tonic-clonic status epilepticus is the most lethal form of this disorder, but even this potentially dangerous type can usually be managed without any permanent injury to the patient if appropriate therapy is instituted within minutes or even hours after the first signs of the status epilepticus are observed (see Chapter 13). If generalized tonic-clonic status epilepticus is not treated appropriately, the patient can suffer damage in several body systems and die as a result of those injuries. The outlook is not so grim for absence status epilepticus, but intellectual function may be affected in some individuals if the seizure activity is allowed to persist for hours or days [39]. Brain metabolism is increased greatly during status epilepticus of any sort [43]. This is especially dangerous in the tonic-clonic form, because the demand for oxygen in the brain is increased at the same time that the seizure disorder is causing protracted or recurrent apneic periods. These two factors increase the likelihood of anoxic brain damage [43]. Compounding the brain's metabolic problems during status epilepticus is the breakdown in cerebral autoregulation that also occurs [43]. Blood flow is inappropriately shunted away from areas that are sensitive to ischemia, and the resistance of the entire cerebrovascular system to systemic hypotension is reduced.

Systemic problems observed in tonic-clonic status epilepticus include cardiac arrhythmias and neurogenic pulmonary edema [43]. The risks of vertebral fractures and torn ligaments that attend any generalized tonic-clonic seizure are exaggerated with protracted or recurrent seizures. With persistent tonic and tonic-clonic seizure activity, substantial muscle injury may occur. This, in turn, causes the release of myoglobin into the bloodstream and clearance of the myoglobin through the kidneys. Substantial myoglobin accumulations in the tubules of the kidney can produce renal failure. Hyperthermia may also develop with protracted status epilepticus. Appropriate treatment can prevent all these complications.

REFERENCES

1. Theodore, W.H., Schulman, E.A., Porter, R.J. Intractable seizures: long-term follow-up after prolonged inpatient treatment in an epilepsy unit. *Epilepsia* 24(3):336–343, 1983.
2. Gastaut, H., Gastaut, J.L., Goncalves e Silva, G.E., et al. Relative frequency of different types of epilepsy: a study employing the classification of the International League Against Epilepsy. *Epilepsia* 16:457–461, 1975.
3. Commission on Classification and Terminology of the International League Against Epilepsy: Proposal for the revised clinical and electroencephalographic classification of epileptic seizures. *Epilepsia* 22:489–501, 1981.
4. Gastaut, H. Clinical and electroencephalographical classification of epileptic seizures. *Epilepsia* 11:102, 1970.
5. Delgado-Escueta, A.V., Treiman, D.M., Walsh, G.O. The treatable epilepsies (part 1). *N. Engl. J. Med.* 308(25):1508–1514, 1983.
6. Asconape, J., Penry, J.K. Some clinical and EEG aspects of benign juvenile myoclonic epilepsy. *Epilepsia* 25(1):108–114, 1984.
7. Meencke, H.J., Janz, D. Neuropathological findings in primary generalized epilepsy: a study of eight cases. *Epilepsia* 25(1):8–21, 1984.
8. Rapin, I. *Children with Brain Dysfunction. Neurology, Cognition, Language, and Behavior.* New York: Raven Press, 1982, p. 284.
9. Rodin, E.A. *The Prognosis of Patients with Epilepsy.* Springfield, Ill.: Charles C Thomas, Publishers, 1968, pp. 455.
10. Goldensohn, E.S., Koehle, R. *EEG Interpretation.* Mt. Kisco, N.Y.: Futura Publishing Co., 1975.

11. Goldensohn, E.S.   The classification of epileptic seizures. In Tower, D.B. (ed.), *The Nervous System,* vol. 2. New York: Raven Press, 1975, p. 261.
12. Sato, S., Dreifuss, F.E., Penry, J.K., et al.   Long-term follow-up of absence seizures. *Neurology* (N.Y.) 33:1590–1595, 1983.
13. Jennings, M.T., Bird, T.D.   Genetic influences in the epilepsies. *Am. J. Dis. Child.* 135:450–457, 1981.
14. Lombroso, C.T.   A prospective study of infantile spasms: clinical and therapeutic correlations. *Epilepsia* 24(2):135–158, 1983.
15. Ellenberg, J.H., Hirtz, D.G., Nelson, K.B.   Age at onset of seizures in young children. *Ann. Neurol.* 15(2):127–134, 1984.
16. Lund, M., Reintoft, H., Simonsen, N.   En kontrollerot social og psykologisk undersogelse af patienter med juvenil myoklon epilepsi. *Ugeskr. Laeger* 137:2415–2418, 1975.
17. Schomer, D.L.   Partial epilepsy. *N. Engl. J. Med.* 309(9):536–539, 1983.
18. Waxman, S.G., Geschwind, N.   The interictal behavior syndrome of temporal lobe epilepsy. *Arch. Gen. Psychiatry* 32:1580–1586, 1975.
19. Blumer, D.   Temporal lobe epilepsy and its psychiatric significance. In Benson, D.F., Blumer, D. (eds.), *Psychiatric Aspects of Neurologic Disease.* New York: Grune & Stratton, 1975, p. 171.
20. Delgado-Escueta, A.V., Treiman, D.M., Walsh, G.O.   The treatable epilepsies (part 2). *N. Engl. J. Med.* 308(26):1576–1584, 1983.
21. Hecker, A., Andermann, F., Rodin, E.A.   Spitting automatism in temporal lobe seizures. *Epilepsia* 13:767, 1972.
22. Goldensohn, E.S., Gold, A.P.   Prolonged behavioral disturbances as ictal phenomena. *Neurology* (N.Y.) 10:1, 1959.
23. Remillard, G.M., Andermann, F., Gloor, P., et al.   Water-drinking as ictal behavior in complex partial seizures. *Neurology* (N.Y.) 31:117, 1981.
24. Flor-Henry, P.   Ictal and interictal psychiatric manifestations in epilepsy: specific or non-specific? *Epilepsia* 13:773, 1972.
25. Babb, R., Eckman, P.B.   Abdominal epilepsy. *J.A.M.A.* 222:65, 1972.
26. Mulder, D.W., Daly, D.   Psychiatric symptoms associated with lesions of temporal lobe. *J.A.M.A.* 150:173, 1952.
27. Slater, E., Beard, A.W.   The schizophrenia-like psychoses of epilepsy: I. Psychiatric aspects. *Br. J. Psychiatry* 109:95, 1963.
28. Mohan, K.J., Salo, M.W., Nagaswami, S.   A case of limbic system dysfunction with hypersexuality and fugue state. *Dis. Nerv. Syst.* 36:621, 1975.
29. McLachlan, R.S., Blume, W.T.   Isolated fear in complex partial status epilepticus. *Ann. Neurol.* 8:639, 1980.
30. Rodin, E.A.   Psychosocial management of patients with complex partial seizures. *Adv. Neurol.* 11:383, 1975.
31. Malamud, N.   Psychiatric disorder with intracranial tumors of the limbic system. *Arch. Neurol.* 17:113, 1967.
32. Gunn, J.   Violence and epilepsy. *N. Engl. J. Med.* 306:298–299, 1982.
33. Mayeux, R., Brandt, J., Rosen, J., et al.   Interictal memory and language impairment in temporal lobe epilepsy. *Neurology* (N.Y.) 30:120, 1980.
34. Booker, H.E.   Management of the difficult patient with complex partial seizures. *Adv. Neurol.* 11:369, 1975.
35. Waxman, S.G., Geschwind, N.   Hypergraphia in temporal lobe epilepsy. *Neurology* (N.Y.) 24:629, 1974.
36. Jackson, J.H.   On epilepsy and epileptiform convulsions. In Taylor, J. (ed.), *Selected Writings of John Hughlings Jackson,* vol. 1. London: Hodder and Stoughton, 1931.
37. Stevens, J.R.   Psychosis and epilepsy. *Ann. Neurol.* 14(3):347–348, 1983.

38. Dana-Haeri, J., Richens, A.   Effect of norethisterone on seizures associated with menstruation. *Elpilepsia* 24(3):377–381, 1983.
39. Ballenger, C.E., III, King, D.W., Gallagher, B.B.   Partial complex status epilepticus. *Neurology* (Cleveland) 33(12):1545–1552, 1983.
40. Niedermeyer, E., Fineyre, F., Riley, T., et al.   Absence status (petit mal status) with focal characteristics. *Arch. Neurol.* 36:417, 1979.
41. Lechtenberg, R.   *The Psychiatrist's Guide to Diseases of the Nervous System.* New York: John Wiley & Sons, 1982.
42. Doose, H., Volzke, E.   Petit mal status in early childhood and dementia. *Neuropadiatrie* 10:10–14, 1979.
43. Engel, J., Jr., Troupin, A.S., Crandall, P.H., et al.   Recent developments in the diagnosis and therapy of epilepsy. *Ann. Intern. Med.* 97:584–598, 1982.

3. Pseudoseizures

Pseudoseizures are episodes that intentionally or incidentally resemble sei-zures. Some physicians divide pseudoseizures into factitious seizures and sei-zure-like phenomena, but most use the terms *pseudoseizure* and *factitious seizure* synonymously. Factitious seizures are episodes of altered behavior purposely contrived to make it appear that the person is having a seizure. Patients who have epilepsy may also have factitious seizures, and so simply determining that a patient has epilepsy does not confirm that the observed seizure activity is authentic. In some cases, individuals in whom epilepsy has been diagnosed and who have received treatment for years prove to have factitious seizures. Which of the patients in whom epilepsy has been diagnosed actually have factitious seizures is difficult to know, because the evaluation of individuals who experience episodes resembling seizures is highly variable.

FACTITIOUS SEIZURES

From 5 to 36 percent of the patients treated as epileptic have factitious seizures rather than, or as well as, true seizures [1, 2]. Most factitious seizures are contrived to gain attention, extract sympathy, or avoid participating in some kind of activity. Whatever the motivation or setting for the contrived seizure, the advantage of having it invariably reduces to providing an escape from a difficult situation or placing the "victim" in an advantageous position [3].

This contrived behavior would provide little secondary gain if it could be recognized, but determining the authenticity of a seizure is difficult, even when the observer is familiar with epilepsy [2]. Experienced neurologists can identify factitious seizures in only 75 percent of cases [4]. Factitious seizures may occur any time after infancy in either male or female patients, but they are more common in adults, especially women [1, 4, 5]. These episodes usually appear first when the patient is between 22 and 32 years old and occur more commonly in individuals who have, or whose families have, obvious psychiatric problems, which are often manifest as severe depression, suicide attempts, and sexual disorders [1, 5–7]. The mean age at which the pseudoseizures first appear is much later than that for most idiopathic epilepsies, but this cannot be used as an indication that the episodes probably are factitious. Most factitious seizures actually seem to be symptomatic seizures, because many of the patients with factitious seizures claim they started after a head injury or severe illness [1]. Patients with factitious seizures usually will provide more etiologic factors in their histories than the patient with true seizures [1]. This wealth of possible etiologies should heighten the physician's level of suspicion, but it is not a sufficient reason to withhold treatment from a patient with possible seizures.

Psychological Features of the Patient

Although these attacks are routinely called *hysterical seizures* or *conversion reactions*, hysteria and psychoses do not play a substantial part in the development of factitious seizures [4]. It is true, however, that patients who experience these episodes have fairly obvious emotional problems (Table 3–1) [1]. Patients with pseudoseizures more often have a history of psychiatric referrals and psychiatric hospitalizations than do patients with authentic epilepsy. They tend to be manipulative and exhibit unusual thought patterns on formal neuropsychological testing. They are highly suggestible and may have factitious seizures with no more provocation than hypnosis or a saline injection.

Their personality profiles exhibit patterns frequently seen in patients with the conversion form of hysteria [1]. They have more difficulties in early family relationships and less ability to cope with their so-called seizure disorder, and

Table 3–1.
Psychological Traits of Patients with Pseudoseizures

Highly suggestible and manipulative
Impaired on neuropsychologic tests
Personality profile suggesting conversion form of hysteria
MMPI revealing unusual thought patterns
Sexual exploitation in childhood common in affected women
History of psychiatric hospitalization in many
Multiple etiologies suggested by patient

they are more concerned with establishing relationships with their physicians than are patients with true seizures [1]. Many of the affected women have histories of sexual exploitation in childhood or adolescence [7]. Both the men and the women have a higher-than-expected incidence of real neurologic problems [1]. In fact, these patients often are somewhat physically or intellectually impaired, and that physical or intellectual impairment may contribute to their lack of adaptability. At some level, they may rely on their factitious seizure disorder to conceal their real inabilities. Rather than exhibiting a mild dementia that normal relationships and responsibilities would quickly reveal, the patient may hide behind the contrived limitations imposed by the seizure disorder.

Clinical Features of Factitious Seizures

The spectrum of behavior exhibited by people with factitious seizures is somewhat limited, and this may help others recognize what is not an authentic seizure. Deciding what is factitious is of more than just academic interest. No one without epilepsy should be exposed to the risks of antiepileptic drugs, but patients with factitious seizures are usually taking several of these agents, because their seizures are inordinately refractory to conventional approaches. In addition, many people with contrived seizures need psychiatric help to develop less destructive techniques for dealing with conflicts and responsibilities. Most factitious seizures actually are easily identified, because the medically unsophisticated patient generally has inaccurate notions of how a seizure should look. Distinguishing the real from the contrived seizures is much more difficult in the patient with well-established epilepsy. Even electroencephalographic monitoring of the episode may fail to reveal the true nature of the attack in patients with chronically abnormal electroencephalographic patterns.

Behavior in factitious seizures tends to be fairly simple and stereotyped [6]. Even in different cultures and historical periods, the similarity of clinical phenomena during the contrived episodes is striking. One hundred years ago, movements suggesting animal activity were relatively common; now, asymmetrical thrashing limb movements are more typical of factitious seizures. Grimacing often occurs, and posturing of the limbs or trunk, trembling, limb jerking, and limb flailing are the most common movements exhibited [6].

In more than 80 percent of cases, there are abnormal limb or trunk movements during the episode [6]. Many patients also experience choking or panic-like states [1]. Seventy percent complain of nausea, cramps, abdominal pain, or disagreeable tastes, and 75 percent have no response or bizarre responses to verbal stimuli during their contrived seizures [6]. Approximately one-third exhibit a change in their breathing patterns, and nearly half will speak, grunt, moan, sob, cough, hum, or make similar noises [6]. Semipurposeful behavior is evident in more than half [6].

Before, during, or after the factitious seizure, patients routinely complain of dizziness, head pain, visual changes, feelings of depersonalization, hot flashes, auditory changes, and other less easily described total body changes. Violent behavior is rare, but the patient may run, cry, chew, or make obscene gestures [6]. The most dramatic features of most factitious seizures are emotional outbursts, acting out, or withdrawal from contact with the environment. These phenomena routinely develop more slowly, appear more labored, and last longer than similar phenomena occurring in true seizures [1].

The unsophisticated patient may be unresponsive for several minutes during a lengthy pseudoseizure but exhibit no postictal phase and abruptly return to normal mentation when the limb and body movements stop [3]. Many patients smile during or immediately after the pseudoseizure, a response not at all typical of true seizures [1]. The patient usually suffers no injuries, and only the most sophisticated patient will urinate during one of these episodes to make it appear more authentic. Most will push away painful stimuli and resist any efforts to interfere with their breathing during all phases of the pseudoseizure [3].

Despite its limitations, the electroencephalograph is a powerful tool in uncovering factitious seizures. Repeatedly normal records obtained at about the time of the apparent seizures, even if they ae not obtained during the seeming ictus, are compelling evidence of a contrived seizure disorder. The electroencephalogram does not usually return to normal immediately after a seizure, except in some generalized absence seizures, and even in these cases the patient often has spike–and–slow wave complexes when seizures are not occurring. During the interictal period, the electroencephalogram will be abnormal in approximately 90 percent of truly epileptic individuals if several records are obtained from the patient [3]. Sleep or hyperventilation will increase the yield of observed abnormalities in patients with true seizure disorders. Photic stimulation and special electrode placement also help to uncover abnormal brain wave activity in the interictal period in patients with epilepsy. Repeatedly normal records, despite such provocative measures, are highly suggestive of a factitious seizure disorder. The use of continuous video and electroencephalographic monitoring allows the physician to record several spontaneous episodes of seizure activity and helps determine whether any of the seizure activity is real [1, 2]

Individuals with Epilepsy and Factitious Seizures

Five to 20 percent of patients with poorly controlled seizures of any type have both factitious and true seizures [2, 4]. That the patient profits in some way from the contrived seizures usually is fairly obvious, but this fact alone does not prove that the episodes are contrived. An electroencephalogram obtained during the pseudoseizure usually is helpful in determining whether the seizure is factitious, but if the background brain wave activity is already abnormal, the electroencephalogram may not prove that the seizure is contrived.

The most reliable technique for evaluating the patient with epilepsy and persistent seizures that may be factitious is simultaneous video and continuous electroencephalographic monitoring [2]. Individual episodes and the electrical changes associated with them can be scrutinized with this long-term monitoring. However, most hospitals are not equipped to observe patients in this way. In the future, less ambiguous evaluation of the seizures may be possible with special techniques, such as positron emission tomography and physiologic studies using nuclear magnetic resonance, that currently are only rarely available. Without objective measures of the seizure's authenticity, the physician is obliged to err on the side of caution and treat patients with questionable episodes.

Contrived seizures occasionally develop in relatives of patients with epilepsy. Some children, for amusement or attention, imitate the seizures they see in their parents or siblings [8]. The parents of children with seizures generally do not behave in this way. Because close relatives of patients with epilepsy are at higher risk of developing seizures than is the general population, any seizures occurring in siblings or children of affected individuals must be considered authentic until proved otherwise [9].

SEIZURE-LIKE PHENOMENA

Alterations in consciousness, perception, or behavior occur in several disorders other than epilepsy (Table 3–2). Most of these are not factitious, some are not neurologic disorders, and many, both neurologic and nonneurologic, are treatable. For most patients, antiepileptic medication is ineffective and inappropriate. These seizure-like phenomena occur in individuals of both sexes and at all ages.

Several phenomena that occur in infants and children are easily confused with epilepsy. These behavioral abnormalities often appear to involve choking or respiratory distress and occasionally occur only during sleep. Vascular problems, such as migraine, account for some of these childhood disorders, but in many cases the disorder is rooted in problems in the relationship between the child and its parents. Electroencephalograms are especially helpful in determining which of these transient phenomena are signs of epilepsy.

Table 3–2.
Seizure-like Phenomena

Jitteriness	Night terrors
Esophageal reflux	Bruxism
Breath-holding spells	Cataplexy
Somnambulism	Migraine
Somniloquy	Psychoses

Brain waves may change during these seizure-like episodes, but typical seizure activity, such as spikes, sharp waves, or bursts of slow waves, do not occur. Electroencephalographic abnormalities may be incidental findings, but this is very rare. With some disorders, such as sleep-related phenomena, the age of the patient at which the signs and symptoms occur is helpful in determining the etiology of the episodic disorder. That the patient responds to antiepileptic medication is not helpful in distinguishing between seizure disorders and seizure-like phenomena, because some seizure-like phenomena respond to specific antiepileptic drugs and others remit coincidentally when medications are given.

Jitteriness

Some newborns and very young infants have paroxysms of shuddering or tremulous movements that are reminiscent of seizures. Identifying seizures in patients of this age is especially difficult, because the immature nervous system produces fairly unique signs when the brain is disturbed by epileptic activity (see Chapter 5). The infant with jitteriness has paroxysmal tremors without any obvious disturbance of consciousness. It may be impossible to ascertain whether the newborn child has altered consciousness, but with electroencephalographic recordings, one can determine whether seizures are responsible for the tremors [10]. Even without using an electroencephalogram, the episodes may be recognized as a movement, rather than a seizure, disorder if the infant has no abnormalities of gaze or eye movements and if the attacks are easily precipitated by a loud noise, flash of light, sudden pain, or abrupt change in position [10]. Also, the tremulous movements in infants with jitteriness usually stop when the affected limb is flexed, a response not seen when the limb movements are related to seizures. Limb movements in most newborns with seizures appear as posturing or irregular jerks. That the infant has jitteriness, rather than seizures, does not mean that the infant has no nervous system damage. Jitteriness often appears in children with hypoxic or ischemic encephalopathy or metabolic problems, such as hypoglycemia, hypocalcemia, or drug withdrawal [10].

Esophageal Reflux

Some infants at 6 to 8 weeks of age suffer episodes of choking, during which they seem to have difficulty breathing [11]. This develops without vomiting, and it is frequently associated with posturing of the arms and legs. The infant may assume an opisthotonic posture and develop cyanosis. This generally occurs in infants who have poor feeding patterns and who must cry for lengthy intervals to get parental attention. Usually, reflux of food into the child's esophagus occurs simultaneously with altered breathing and posturing. Increased physical contact between the parent and the child may eliminate this behavior.

Breath Holding

As many as 1 of 20 infants and children have breath-holding spells. Although this is not a specifically hereditary problem, 1 of 4 children who exhibit this behavior has another family member with a history of breath-holding spells. These spells usually first occur at 6 months to 4 years of age. The child stops breathing for several seconds or minutes and becomes cyanotic or pale. In most children, this is a behavioral abnormality associated with protracted anger and frustration. Sometimes, it is associated with vagal reflex abnormalities, but in such cases the behavior abates as the child matures. Other behaviorial eccentricities often develop with maturation if the child is holding his breath in reaction to excessive frustration. This behavior generally is best managed with family therapy rather than with any drugs, since it usually is part of a pathologic family interaction and involves most, if not all, family members.

Shuddering and Dystonia

Abnormal posturing is called *dystonia* when it appears in an individual who is alert and aware of the change acutely appearing in his limbs and trunk. The muscle tone in dystonias often is normal, even when the position assumed appears strained and painful. Paroxysmal dystonias are very rare, but they occur in some hereditary diseases and may even develop from such common neurologic diseases as multiple sclerosis if extensive cerebellar damage is present [12].

The acute onset of the abnormal posture and the quick resolution after seconds or minutes of disturbed limb positions, neck posture, or spinal curvature suggests seizure activity. Contributing to this notion is the apparent usefulness of phenytoin in suppressing some of these paroxysmal dystonias. Electroencephalographic studies will show, however, that cerebral activity is normal during the attack.

Similar doubts about true seizure activity may arise in individuals with other types of paroxysmal movement or postural disorders. Some children have attacks of limb or trunk jerking that last several seconds [13]. The affected individual's consciousness is not impaired, but the suddenness of the movements may precipitate a fall. Many parents describe these as shuddering attacks. This disorder exhibits a familial pattern and is associated with essential tremor, an idiopathic limb movement disorder that often responds to low doses of propranolol hydrochloride. Paroxysmal attacks of shuddering are not eliminated by antiepileptic medications and are not associated with any abnormalities on brain wave recordings [13]. Many of these postural disturbances that are refractory to treatment abate or change with age, but in some cases, they become progressively worse.

Transient Ischemia and Hypotension

Vascular disorders of several types can impair nervous system function transiently by reducing blood flow to the brain. In the elderly, the cause is likely to be a cardiac arrhythmia, whereas in younger people it may develop with emboli originating on damaged heart valves [14]. Valvular heart disease is an especially bothersome cause of transient neurologic deficits, because many of the diseases that cause the valvular damage can also involve the nervous system directly and produce seizures [15]. The patient with systemic lupus erythematosus may have transient ischemic attacks with emboli originating on the vegetations of Libman-Sacks endocarditis or have seizures associated with a lupus cerebritis [16].

With cardiac arrhythmias and embolic disease, the transient neurologic problem may be syncope, but focal neurologic signs, including disorientation and aphasia, can occur [17]. If the attack lasts less than 24 hours, it is, by definition, a transient ischemic attack. If it lasts longer, it is a stroke, even if all the neurologic deficits clear thoroughly. The identification of the cardiac arrhythmia may require nothing more than a Holter monitor recording of cardiac activity over the course of a full day [18]. Recognition of valvular disease is often considerably more complicated, especially when the patient has no murmur or other signs of valvular heart disease. Various types of echocardiography are available for investigation of the valves and should be used if there is reason to suspect embolic disease [19].

Patients with well-treated hypertension may develop syncope or transient ischemic attacks without syncope if antihypertensive medication is more effective than the brain can tolerate [20]. The normal systemic blood pressure achieved with antihypertensive medication may produce hypotensive episodes in the head when minor stresses occur. Narrowing of the major vessels of the head is also a common cause of transient ischemic attacks, but syncope most often occurs with disease in the vertebrobasilar, rather than the carotid, artery system (Fig. 3–1). With impaired blood flow to the brainstem, the patient may develop cranial nerve symptoms, such as double vision, slurred speech, and vertigo, preceding the syncope. Transient ischemic attacks outside the posterior fossa usually produce focal neurologic signs and symptoms, such as aphasia, hemiparesis, visual field cuts, and hemianesthesia, with somewhat altered or even intact consciousness. The management of transient ischemic attacks in either the vertebrobasilar or carotid systems is very controversial.

Some people have altered consciousness associated with specific activities [20]. Coughing or urinating may trigger an exaggerated vasovagal reflex in otherwise normal people, and with spur formation on cervical vertebrae, the vertebral arteries may be compromised when the individual turns his head. Both problems may cause syncope. Pressure over the carotid artery also occasionally induces syncope by provoking a transient bradycardia in susceptible individuals. Much rarer are skeletal anomalies, such as basilar impression, an

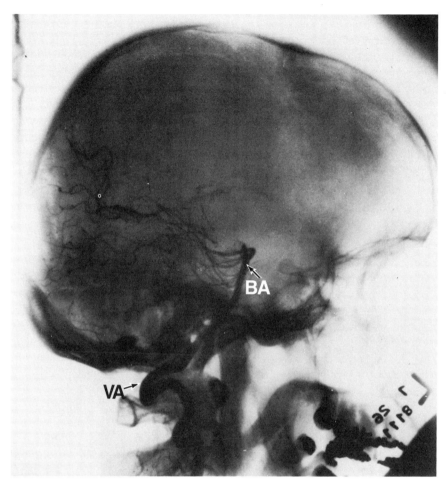

Figure 3–1.
Transient ischemic attacks involving the vertebral (VA) or basilar (BA) arteries can produce episodic losses of consciousness that may resemble seizures.

abnormally formed junction between the skull and the spine, which interfere with the blood supply to the brainstem and cause recurrent attacks of unconsciousness [21].

Metabolic Disorders

Most metabolic disorders are not confused with epilepsy, but some that present with syncope and little else cause diagnostic problems. Transient hypoglycemia is a very rare cause of syncope in individuals not being treated with hypog-

45

lycemic agents, but it does occur with some insulin-secreting tumors and even in the early stages of some cases of diabetes mellitus [22]. Much more common is hyperventilation associated with acute anxiety that causes syncope by inducing a respiratory alkalosis [23]. Because seizures may be precipitated by hyperventilation, an electroencephalogram may be needed to determine whether epilepsy is the basis for the syncope or the hyperventilation alone is responsible. With any metabolic disorder that causes syncope, the underlying disease must be treated to eliminate the cause of the altered consciousness. In cases of hyperventilation, chronic anxiety may underlie the recurrent change in breathing that induces the syncope. Many patients who hyperventilate profit from psychiatric intervention of some type.

Sleep-Related Disorders

Sleepwalking (somnambulism), sleep-talking (somniloquy), and night terrors are not caused by seizure activity, but features of each of these nocturnal phenomena often resemble seizures [24, 25]. Complicating the interpretation of these phenomena is the fact that seizures do occur during sleep and can induce a child or adult to walk or talk or appear acutely frightened. When the problem is epilepsy, the affected individual usually will have seizures when awake and exhibit other signs of abnormal brain activity, such as generalized convulsions, postictal confusion, and premonitory auras. Even with epilepsy types that characteristically start with sleep-related seizures, such as benign juvenile myoclonic epilepsy, the seizures eventually will occur while the patient is awake.

With both seizures and sleep-related phenomena, the affected individual generally has no recall of the abnormal behavior when he or she is fully awake [26]. The confusion, irritability, and combativeness exhibited by some people during these episodes support the notion that epilepsy is responsible, but an electroencephalogram will establish that epilepsy is not involved [24]. Electroencephalographic recordings during sleep will establish the nature of the episodes when there is a question about their benign character.

Bruxism (tooth grinding) also arouses concern that a convulsion is occurring, but as an isolated sign it is too common in the general population to warrant investigation [27]. Bed-wetting (enuresis) justifies more concern, even though it is also a benign sleep phenomenon in young children; in adults, it may be a sign of nocturnal seizures [24].

Cataplexy

Some patients with narcolepsy, a form of hypersomnia, develop cataplexy, sleep paralysis, and hallucinations [28]. The cataplexy is a sudden loss of tone and posture that may cause dangerous falls [29] The acute attacks usually occur with excitment or stress and are very much like generalized myoclonic seizures in their brevity and intensity [30].

Sleep paralysis is a transient loss of voluntary movements just after awakening. This may persist for several seconds before the terrified individual can get up. If there is no history of sleep attacks, this transient paralysis is easily confused with postictal weakness (Todd paralysis). Contributing to a misdiagnosis of epilepsy in narcoleptic individuals are the hypnagogic and hypnopompic hallucinations also associated with narcolepsy. These are vivid images or sounds that appear as the affected person is falling asleep or awakening.

These problems occur in a variety of combinations, but the most common element for any individual with cataplexy, hallucinations, or sleep paralysis is the sleep attack [29]. The sleep attacks will suggest narcolepsy rather than epilepsy, and nonepileptic electroencephalographic patterns during these various neurologic phenomena will help establish the correct diagnosis.

Migraine

Migraine headaches are fundamentally a vascular disorder rather than a specifically neurologic one, but they can cause disorientation, memory disturbances, and personality changes when they occur in either children or adults. The characteristic pain and a family history of migraine usually simplify the identification of this problem. The electroencephalogram obtained during a migraine attack usually will be abnormal, and so this becomes a less useful diagnostic tool.

Complicating the diagnosis of migraine are the aura that may precede the attacks and the focal neurologic signs that may occur with some attacks. The aura may be a poorly formed visual hallucination or a gastrointestinal complaint. Especially worrisome are basilar migraines. In these, the basilar artery is involved and symptoms include vertigo, gait disorders, double vision, and vomiting. The onset of basilar migraines is typically later in life than that for idiopathic seizures, whereas classic migraines often develop at about puberty. Basilar migraine also causes electroencephalographic abnormalities, including spikes in the occipital region. A trial period of medicating the patient to suppress the migraine headache is often the simplest way to determine if this disorder is responsible for the patient's symptoms.

Psychoses

Although there is a common tendency to overstate the problem, there are some psychiatric disorders that are exceedingly difficult to distinguish from seizure disorders [31]. Especially in psychoses with transient cognitive or affective disorders, the patient may appear fairly normal between attacks and claim little recall of behavior during the attack. As in epilepsy, the pattern of signs and symptoms over the course of months often helps to establish the nature of the problem. All such recurrent psychiatric problems should be investigated for possible neurologic or endocrinologic bases, but in most cases the pattern of the disorder will belie its psychiatric basis.

REFERENCES

1. Wilkus, R.J., Dodrill, C.B., Thompson, P.M.   Intensive EEG monitoring and psychological studies of patients with pseudoepileptic seizures. *Epilepsia* 25(1):100–107, 1984.
2. Theodore, W.H., Schulman, E.A., Porter, R.J.   Intractable seizures: long-term follow-up after prolonged inpatient treatment in an epilepsy unit. *Epilepsia* 24(3):336–343, 1983.
3. Massey, E.W., Riley, T.L.   Pseudoseizures: recognition and treatment. *Psychosomatics* 21:987, 1980.
4. King, D.W., Gallagher, B.B., Marvin, A.J., et al.   Pseudoseizures: diagnostic evaluation. *Neurology* (N.Y.) 32:18–23, 1982.
5. Roy, A.   Hysterical seizures. *Arch. Neurol.* 36:447, 1979.
6. Gulick, T.A., Spinks, I.P., King, D.W.   Pseudoseizures: ictal phenomena. *Neurology* (N.Y.) 32:24–30, 1982.
7. La Barbera, J.D., Dozier, J.E.   Hysterical seizures: the role of exploitation. *Psychosomatics* 21:897, 1980.
8. Lechtenberg, R.   *Epilepsy and The Family.* Cambridge, Mass.: Harvard University Press, 1984.
9. Jennings, M.T., Bird, T.D.   Genetic influences in the epilepsies. *Am. J. Dis. Child.* 135:450–457, 1981.
10. Volpe, J.J.   Neonatal seizures. *Clin. Perinoatol.* 4(1):43–63, 1977.
11. Cohen, S.   Motor disorders of the esophagus. *N. Engl. J. Med.* 301:184, 1979.
12. Gilman, S., Bloedel, J., Lechtenberg, R.   *Disorders of The Cerebellum.* Philadelphia: F.A. Davis Co., 1981.
13. Vanasse, M., Bedard, P., Andermann, F.   Shuddering attacks in children: an early manifestation of essential tremor. *Neurology* (N.Y.) 26:1027–1030, 1976.
14. Beal, M.F., Williams, R.S., Richardson, E.P., Jr., et al.   Cholesterol embolism as a cause of transient ischemic attacks and cerebral infarction. *Neurology* (N.Y.) 31:860, 1981.
15. Ueda, K., Toole, J.F., McHenry, L.C., Jr.   Carotid and vertebrobasilar transient ischemic attacks: clinical and angiographic correlation. *Neurology* (N.Y.) 29:1094–1101, 1979.
16. Fox, Y.S., Spence, A.M., Wheelis, R.F., Healey, L.A.   Cerebral embolism in Libman-Sacks endocarditis. *Neurology* (N.Y.) 30:487–491, 1980.
17. Toole, J.F., Yuson, C.P.   Transient ischemic attacks with normal arteriograms: serious or benign prognosis. *Ann. Neurol.* 1:100–102, 1977.
18. Wolf, P.A., Dauber, T.R., Thomas, H.E.J., Kannel, W.B.   Epidemiological assessment of chronic atrial fibrillation and stroke: the Framingham study. *Neurology* (N.Y.) 28:973–977, 1978.
19. Knopman, D.S., Anderson, D.C., Asinger, R.W., et al.   Indications for echocardiography in patients with ischemic stroke. *Neurology* (N.Y.) 32(9):1005–1012, 1982.
20. Hickler, R.G.   Orthostatic hypotension and syncope. *N. Engl. J. Med.* 296:336, 1977.

21. Taylor, A.R., Chakravorty, B.C.   Clinical syndromes associated with basilar impression. *Arch. Neurol.* 10:475, 1964.
22. Hypoglycaemia and personality. *Br. Med. J.* 2:134, 1974.
23. Booker, H.E.   Management of the difficult patient with complex partial seizures. *Adv. Neurol.* 11:369, 1975.
24. Hartmann, E.   Sleep. In Nicholi, A.M. (ed.). *The Harvard Guide to Modern Psychiatry.* Cambridge, Mass.: Belknap Press, 1978, p. 103.
25. Pedley, T.A., Guilleminault, C.   Episodic nocturnal wanderings. Response to anticonvulsant drug therapy. *Ann. Neurol.* 2:30, 1977.
26. Karacan, I., Moore, C.A., Williams, R. L.   The narcoleptic syndrome. *Psychiatr. Ann.* 9:69, 1979.
27. Hartmann, E.   Alcohol and bruxism. *N. Engl. J. Med.* 301:333, 1979.
28. Zarcone, V.   Narcolepsy. *N. Engl. J. Med.* 288:1156, 1973.
29. Guilleminault, C., Wilson, R.A., Dement, W.C.   A study on cataplexy. *Arch. Neurol.* 31:255, 1974.
30. Schacter, M., Parkes, J.D.   Fluvoxamine and clomipramine in the treatment of cataplexy. *J. Neurol. Neurosurg. Psychiatry* 43:171, 1980.
31. Lechtenberg, R.   *The Psychiatrist's Guide to Diseases of The Nervous System.* New York: John Wiley & Sons, 1982.

4. Origin of Seizures

There are many different diseases and disorders that cause seizures. These include central nervous system disease, systemic problems that affect the nervous system, hereditary defects in brain development, and scores of poorly defined metabolic and membrane disturbances. By definition, unexplained— that is, idiopathic—seizures cannot be traced to a defect or deficiency in the brain or elsewhere. Implicit in this designation is the understanding that with better diagnostic techniques fewer seizures will be idiopathic [1]. Even when the epilepsy is presumed to be symptomatic rather than idiopathic, follow-up may reveal that the seizures and the problem thought to underlie the seizures are actually unrelated. For any patient, all that can be established is the probable cause of the seizures and, hence, of the epilepsy.

Characteristics of the patient and the seizures help limit the spectrum of probable causes. Young patients are at higher risk for certain types of disorders than are older patients. In newborns, birth asphyxia and hereditary metabolic problems often cause seizures. In children, head injuries and nervous system infections are a more common basis for seizures, and in the adult who develops epilepsy at 40 or 50 years of age, the likelihood that a brain tumor underlies the seizure disorder is high. The character and causes of epilepsy in infancy and childhood generally are very different from those of the adult and will be discussed separately (see Chapter 5).

Seizures in any age group that are initially well controlled and later recur despite therapeutic antiepileptic drug levels are often a result of structural

Table 4–1.
Causes of Epilepsy In Adults

Trauma	Vascular inflammation
Infection	Parasites
Stroke	Poisons
Hemorrhage	Drugs
Tumor	Idiopathic epilepsy
Vascular malformation	

brain damage. That structural problem may be a tumor or abscess in the brain, a blood clot overlying the brain, a vasculitis or vascular malformation in the head, or a cerebral contusion [2]. Periodic reevaluation of the patient with idiopathic seizures will uncover unsuspected lesions in some patients.

Signs and symptoms associated with seizures often help to elucidate the basis of the neurologic problem (Table 4–1) [1, 3]. A rapidly progressive paralysis or receptive aphasia associated with an ear infection suggests a brain abscess extending from the inflammation in the ear. Children with café au lait spots, ash leaf spots, or port-wine nevi are at high risk of having nervous system tumors associated with these dermatologic signs of hereditary developmental disorders. Adults with unilateral headaches and audible bruits over the head may have arteriovenous malformations in or overlying the brain. Any focal neurologic signs or systemic disorders occurring in conjunction with the seizures should be considered to be related to the epilepsy until enough evidence is gathered to prove they are not.

IDIOPATHIC EPILEPSY

Most seizures develop for no apparent reason [1]. This is especially true of generalized absence (petit mal) seizures and the majority of complex partial seizures. Generalized tonic-clonic seizures may appear after head trauma or a central nervous system infection, but they, too, usually develop without any antecedent injury or infection. Presumably, the cause of idiopathic seizures is at the level of nerve cell organization or interactions. Supporting this idea are an increasing number of histologic studies of brains from patients who had idiopathic epilepsy.

Diffuse developmental abnormalities are clearly present in the brains of some people with generalized epilepsies [4]. This brain dysgenesis involves little more than abnormal migration or orientation of nerve cells in the cortex of many of the patients studied [4]. Patients with complex partial seizures originating in temporal lobe foci may have microscopic changes in nerve cell density and associated changes in the glial supporting tissue on the inner face of the temporal lobe. This is called *mesial temporal sclerosis* and is assumed to occur after ischemic, hypoxic, or other damage to this part of the brain.

Whether it is the cause of, result of, or incidental finding with seizures is uncertain.

Since the diagnosis of diffuse developmental abnormalities requires examination of an autopsy or biopsy specimen, most epilepsies caused by microscopic structural lesions will be considered idiopathic until the patient dies or has surgery. In many cases, pathologic examination of the brain of an individual who had lifelong epilepsy will reveal no abnormalities that could account for the seizure disorder. Because much of the brain's activity is inhibitory, it is likely that impaired function in one part of the brain could allow abnormal activity, such as seizure activity, to develop in another part of the brain.

The notion that damage to the brain occurs before or at birth in patients with idiopathic seizures has been popular for several decades, but it has not yet been proved. Some of the ischemic or hypoxic changes in the brains of patients with idiopathic epilepsy may be caused by long-term seizure activity or even long-term antiepileptic drug treatment, but this, too, is still uncertain. With the development of new investigative tools, such as positron emission tomography and nuclear magnetic resonance, further pathologic bases for epilepsy will be defined and fewer seizure disorders will be considered idiopathic.

TRAUMATIC BRAIN DAMAGE

Brain damage from head injuries is common in both children and adults, whether male or female. Head injuries resulting from automobile accidents alone are a major public health problem, but added to these are head injuries sustained in falls, sporting accidents, industrial mishaps, and child abuse. Most of these are preventable. Head injuries in automobile accidents usually occur because no protective restraints, such as seat belts, air bags, or infant seats, are used. Sporting injuries can be minimized by protective head gear. Industrial head trauma has abated considerably since hard hats have been worn as standard equipment on construction sites. Injuries associated with child abuse can only be stopped by protecting the child from assault.

With any head injury, the initial assessment of the patient will determine whether hospitalization is necessary and whether complications, such as epilepsy, are likely to ensue. The severity of the trauma and the social circumstances of the patient must be considered in determining the level and duration of follow-up. A child with fairly mild injuries but with a history of multiple injuries may require hospitalization until the safety of the home environment can be adequately assessed. The risk of seizure activity after the trauma usually plays only a small role in determining whether the patient will be hospitalized, because seizures can occur days, months, or years after head trauma. Despite the delay in their onset, these seizures may still be symptomatic of the injuries sustained with the trauma [1]. The risk of late seizure activity does correlate with the patient's initial appearance and deficits, but no patient with severe head trauma can be assured that seizures will never occur simply because they do not occur within a few months of the injury [5].

Young infants face special risks, because the bones of the skull are not fused and the fontanelles are large enough to allow direct injury to the brain with a well-directed blow. Some cultures still practice molding of the infant's head by tightly binding the skull, which can inadvertently cause trauma to the poorly protected brain of the infant.

Because the adult skull is fairly rigid, a fracture of the cranial vault indicates that the blow to the head was substantial and a brain injury is likely to have occurred. This convenient, though not very reliable, measure of the head trauma is not available when assessing head trauma in infants. The plasticity of the infant skull allows the brain to sustain massive trauma without leaving telltale fractures in the overlying skull. Even in adults, fractures may occur but be inapparent. Basilar skull fractures and injuries to the cribriform plate (under the frontal lobes) are especially difficult to detect even with tomographic studies of the regions. Any discharge of blood mixed with spinal fluid from the nose or ears must be assumed to be from a skull fracture, even when none appears on a skull roentgenogram. Patients with these types of occult skull fractures are at high risk of developing a posttraumatic meningitis. The subarachnoid space is seeded with bacteria from the sinuses or from the middle ear. If the patient develops seizures within a few days of an injury that produces cerebrospinal fluid otorrhea or rhinorrhea, meningitis must be considered the most probable cause of the seizures.

Posttraumatic Seizures

Seizures occurring within seconds or minutes of head trauma are called *impact seizures,* and these are an indication that at least the transient impact on the brain was substantial. Impact seizures are usually generalized tonic-clonic seizures. Even when a few occur in rapid succession at the time of the injury, they do not indicate that this type of seizure will appear again later or become a chronic problem. When seizures do recur weeks or months after the head injury, they may be either generalized or partial. If the damage involves a fairly limited part of the brain, such as the leading edge of the temporal lobe, the patient often develops partial seizures. Focal motor or focal sensory seizures may appear long after the patient recovers from the injury, but any of the more common types of epilepsy may appear early after the trauma or after a delay of weeks [1, 5].

Posttraumatic epilepsy has different implications depending on whether it occurs early or late. The early form is often a transient problem, whereas the late form is usually a persistent seizure disorder. With early posttraumatic epilepsy, seizures occur during the first week after the injury and are often limited

Table 4–2.
Factors Increasing the Risk of Late Epilepsy

Intracranial hematoma	Posttraumatic amnesia
Early epilepsy	of more than 24
Depressed skull fracture	hours
Dural tear	Focal neurologic signs

to focal motor phenemona, such as a twitching leg or arm; these focal signs do not progress to generalized tonic-clonic seizures [6]. Two-thirds of the patients with early posttraumatic epilepsy do not develop persistent seizure disorders [6].

With late posttraumatic epilepsy, the patient has partial or generalized seizures that persist years after the initial trauma (Table 4–2). This problem is especially likely if the patient has bleeding inside the skull or the brain because of the injury [6]. An even higher risk of late epilepsy attends the patient with a blood clot that must be removed within 2 weeks of the injury. In other words, the likelihood of developing a persistent seizure disorder is lower if the patient has a chronic subdural hematoma rather than an epidural or acute subdural hematoma. Many of the events surrounding the initial trauma give some indication of the risk of late epilepsy. If the patient has early posttraumatic seizures or a depressed skull fracture, the risk is greater [6]. The likelihood of late epilepsy increases substantially if the depressed skull fracture is associated with a tear in the dura mater or if there are focal neurologic signs.

If the patient does not suffer a depressed skull fracture or intracranial hematoma, the risk of late epilepsy is only 1 percent [6]. In patients who have an early seizure, the risk is 22 percent if there was also a posttraumatic amnesia lasting less than 24 hours. With posttraumatic amnesia lasting more than 24 hours, the likelihood that the patient will develop late epilepsy increases to 30 percent [6]. The type and frequency of early seizures does not affect the probability that late epilepsy will develop. Changes in the patient's electroencephalogram early after the head trauma are not helpful in predicting the likelihood of late epilepsy [5].

Postcraniotomy Seizures

Although a craniotomy is not generally viewed as a form of trauma, it is traumatic. In most neurosurgical procedures, the dura mater is cut and damage to the cerebral cortex is unavoidable. The risk of epilepsy after a craniotomy is 20 percent [6]. This risk is lower for procedures in which the dura mater is not opened and higher after procedures in which cortical tissue must be removed. If a cerebral abscess, ruptured middle cerebral artery aneurysm, intracerebral hemorrhage, or arteriovenous malformation is the reason for the craniotomy, the likelihood of postoperative seizures is increased. The risk is also increased if the patient had epilepsy before the surgery or if the first seizure occurs within the first postoperative week [6]. This does not mean that patients who must have neurosurgery will necessarily have a persistent seizure disorder. It does mean that ambiguous neurologic phenomena appearing after intracranial surgery should be managed as epilepsy if they at all resemble seizures.

POSTINFECTIOUS SEIZURES

Several types of diffuse central nervous system infections lower the seizure threshold transiently or permanently and induce partial or generalized seizures. Common bacterial causes include *Hemophilus influenzae* in children, pneumococcal and meningococcal agents in adults, and streptococcal or staphylococcal bacteria in individuals with posttraumatic meningitis. Tuberculosis is still a very common cause of meningitis throughout the world and may produce massive granulomas in the brain in severe cases. Many viral causes of men-

Figure 4–1.
This electroencephalogram was obtained from a 72-year-old woman who had transient episodes of altered behavior for which she was amnesic. These episodes were subsequently associated with generalized tonic-clonic seizures. Her spinal fluid was consistently bloody, but her arteriogram revealed no vascular problem. On her electroencephalogram, there are periodic slow wave discharges (x). She was believed to have a herpetic encephalitis. The seizures were treated with carbamazepine and stopped within 2 weeks.

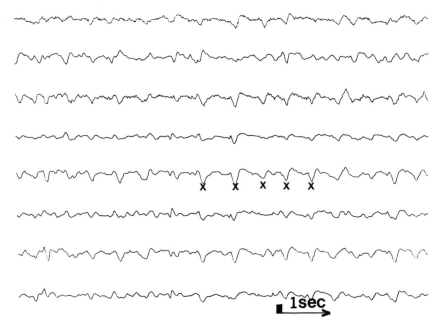

ingoencephalitis leave the patient with epilepsy if he survives the acute infection; *Herpes simplex* often is implicated in these infections (Fig. 4–1). People with poor immune systems are vulnerable to a variety of fungi including *Actinomyces* and *Nocardia,* but survival with these infections is very limited.

With an acute meningitis or encephalitis, many patients will have seizures, but after the infection has resolved, the seizures usually stop. Seizures occur in meningitis because most of these infections are not limited to the meninges. The cerebral cortex is irritated to some extent in all but the mildest meningeal infections, which accounts for the fairly high incidence of seizures in this noncortical problem.

It is difficult to predict in whom the seizures will persist or recur. Whether the infection is bacterial, viral, or fungal plays less of a role in determining which seizures will persist than the focal damage associated with the infection. The type of seizure occurring with the infection may disappear after treatment of the meningoencephalitis, only to be replaced by other types months after the infection. Postinfectious seizures usually are generalized.

PARASITIC INFESTATIONS

Parasites cause much of the epilepsy that occurs in countries with high rates of parasitic infestation. The parasites generally damage the cerebral cortex either by directly invading the brain or by depositing eggs that are trapped in the central nervous system. Cysticercosis from the pork tapeworm *Taenia solium* is especially common in Mexico and often is seen also in people from the Philippines. Schistosomiasis, an infection by a parasite dependent on an intermediate snail host, is widespread in the less industrialized areas of the Orient, and cerebral malaria, the most virulent form this protozoan assumes, is still a frequent cause of acute seizure disorders in tropical countries [7]. Although the parasite may not cause much damage as it invades the brain, immune reactions in the nervous system to the foreign agent may produce a scar that serves as the focus for the seizure activity. Fortunately, control of the seizures developing in people with these parasitic infestations does not depend on eradication of the parasite. Complete seizure control can be achieved with antiepileptic medications, even when irreversible structural damage and viable parasites exist in the brain. Seizures developing with any of these parasitic infestations may be partial or generalized.

BRAIN TUMORS

Seizures appearing in an adult who has suffered no trauma, does not abuse alcohol, and does not have a central nervous system infection are probably from a primary or metastatic brain tumor [8]. These qualifications make this cause of seizures relatively infrequent, simply because trauma, alcoholism, and infections are common causes of epilepsy in adult life. In many patients with brain tumors, focal neurologic signs are associated with seizures, but even when the seizures occur as the only symptom of the neoplasia, the tumor may be highly invasive [3]. The type of tumor is not related to the type of epilepsy that develops, but the location of the tumor may affect whether the seizures are focal or generalized. Metastatic carcinomas and cystic astro-cytomas can precipitate the same seizure types, but tumors in the occipital lobe, whether they are from an astrocytoma or a malignant melanoma, will produce focal sensory seizures with visual hallucinations and a visual field cut. Seizures developing with tumors may be either partial or generalized.

Whether the tumor is removed or left untreated, the seizure disorder initiated by this lesion usually persists and requires antiepileptic treatment. If the tumor cannot be completely removed or arrested, control of the epilepsy may fail as the tumor grows.

Brain tumors rarely cause seizures in children. Of course, there are some notable exceptions, such as those associated with hereditary nervous system diseases in which tumors appear in the cerebrum during the first months of life. Even with these congenital problems, brain malformations rather than tumors are the usual explanation for the seizures in affected children. Most childhood tumors are in the brainstem or the cerebellum, areas that do not evoke seizure activity when damaged [9]. With subarachnoid spread of the tumor cells, substantial cortical irritation can lead to seizures, but this is a relatively late effect of lesions that spread in this way [10].

In both children and adults, what appears to be a tumor on radiographic studies should be biopsied whenever that is feasible. Occasionally, a granuloma or other type of focal inflammation from tuberculosis, parasites, or other agents will masquerade as a mass in the brain.

VASCULAR DISEASE

Aside from the vascular problems that produce signs and symptoms similar to those seen in epilepsy, there are vascular disorders that cause seizures. They may induce this epileptic activity by irritation, ischemia, or irreversible damage in the cerebral cortex, and in most cases, the epilepsy that results does not spontaneously remit. Adults and children of both sexes are susceptible to vascular problems, and, as with tumors, the age of the patient helps limit the spectrum of vascular lesions responsible for the epilepsy. Systemic signs are invaluable in defining epilepsy associated with vasculitis, and persistent neurologic deficits help in the recognition of occlusive and hemorrhagic vascular lesions [8].

Stroke

A stroke is permanent damage to the brain caused by a vascular lesion. The lesion usually is caused by occlusion of or bleeding from an artery or

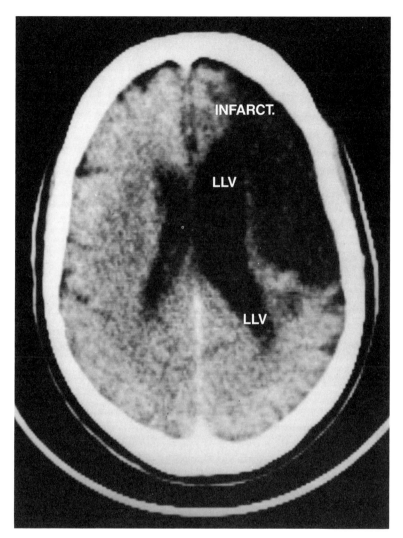

Figure 4–2.
If the patient survives a complete occlusion of the internal carotid artery, his computed
tomogram may look like this after the infarcted brain tissue (INFARCT.) has been
cleared away. This patient had a dense expressive aphasia and a right hemiplegia.
The left lateral ventricle (LLV) is distended because of hydrocephalus ex vacuo, a
compensatory enlargement of the ventricles when cerebral tissue is lost.

vein supplying or draining the brain (Fig. 4–2). With an obstruction, it is irrelevant whether the source of the occlusion is an atherosclerotic plaque in
an artery, hypertensive vascular disease, an embolus from the carotid artery,
or spasm associated with a subarachnoid hemorrhage. Rather, the type
of neurologic problem and the probability of an associated seizure disorder

are determined by the area of the cerebral cortex damaged by the vascular occlusion.

A seizure occurring at the time of the cerebrovascular incident does not help to define the cause of the event. Seizures may occur with bleeding into the subarachnoid space, after cerebral infarction caused by an embolus from a diseased aortic valve, or with an intracerebral hemorrhage from hypertensive vascular disease [11–13]. It has not yet been established whether emboli or hemorrhages are more likely to cause seizures at the time of the acute event. Regardless of whether seizures occur with the initial signs of the stroke, structural damage late in life, from a stroke or from transient cerebral hypoxia, may lead to a seizure focus within weeks or months of the injury [1]. Epilepsy occasionally develops years after the stroke, but this type of neurologic disorder suggests that, as a result of the stroke, the patient has a slightly lowered seizure threshold which has been reached because of systemic problems. With such a lapse of years before the onset of epilepsy, the old vascular injury should not be implicated until other etiologies, such as a metastatic tumor or a meningitis, are eliminated.

Vascular Malformation

Vascular malformations in the brain cause seizures by ischemic injury to the brain around the malformation, as well as by direct injury to cortical tissue from hemorrhages. Within the malformation, the pattern of blood flow is likely to shift as the individual matures, and the resulting changes in cerebral perfusion can be damaging or irritating to the brain, even when the malformation is small [14]. Blood is shunted away from cortex that needs a high volume of blood flow to continue functioning or to maintain its structural integrity. The walls of the malformation often are imperfectly formed and much more vulnerable to rupture than are normal blood vessels. When ischemia and hemorrhage are not problems, the individual with the malformation may still develop epilepsy because of the irritative effect of the malformation as a mass in the head.

Arteritis

With a few diseases that cause arteritis, affected individuals develop seizures. The most common of these diseases is systemic lupus erythematosus, an inflammatory disease that can cause ischemia and seizures in young adults. Central nervous system involvement occurs in 59 percent of patients with systemic lupus erythematosus, and epilepsy is a common sign of this involvement [15]. Patients with lupus are at additional risk of brain damage from emboli originating in the heart on diseased mitral or aortic valves [16]. This complicates the evaluation and treatment of patients with lupus and seizures, because either embolic disease from Libman-Sacks endocarditis or ischemic damage from lupus cerebritis can cause the seizures [16]. Seventeen to 50 percent of patients with systemic lupus erythematosus and central nervous system involvement have seizures [15]. The only other neurologic problem that is as common in patients with lupus is an organic psychosis.

There are many other types of inflammatory vascular disease that affect cranial blood vessels, but with most, the neurologic problem usually seen is stroke rather than epilepsy. Periarteritis nodosa can evoke seizures, but this may be more from hypertensive vascular disease induced by renal involvement than from direct brain involvement. The arteritides of the elderly, such as temporal arteritis and polymyalgia rheumatica, typically do not cause seizures, but they can lead to strokes.

Hypertensive Encephalopathy

Seizures, papilledema, obtundation, and other focal neurologic signs develop abruptly in some individuals, with an acute elevation of their blood pressure. Whether this hypertensive encephalopathy is distinct from other types of cerebrovascular disease is controversial, but it probably is not. Intracerebral bleeding and infarction associated with the hypertension almost certainly precipitate the seizures and obtundation in this condition. As in any stroke, the vascular problems, such as bleeding and hypertension, must be stabilized at the same time that the seizure disorder is investigated and treated.

METABOLIC DISEASE

Abnormal serum electrolyte or glucose levels can trigger seizures in patients with epilepsy and even in people without a chronic seizure disorder [1, 17]. Renal or hepatic failure can also evoke seizures, even when electrolytes are fairly normal, and seizures may recur until these metabolic problems are corrected [1]. Seizures associated with inborn errors of metabolism usually appear early in infancy or childhood, but some first appear in adult life [18].

Most hereditary metabolic diseases that cause epilepsy as a prominent symptom involve the gray matter of the brain much more that the white matter, but there are exceptions. Adrenoleukodystrophy, a recessively inherited, sex-linked, disorder affecting myelinization in the brain, causes electroencephalographic changes early in life and occasionally causes seizures associated with progressive dementia [19]. The gray matter diseases more typically causing epilepsy include Tay-Sachs disease and other types of hexosaminidase deficiency. These are discussed in Chapter 5.

ALCOHOL- AND DRUG-RELATED SEIZURES

Alcoholism and dependence on other drugs can lead to epilepsy by one of several mechanisms. Seizures may develop in the alcoholic individual or the drug addict as a result of head trauma incurred during episodes of intoxication or impaired coordination. Withdrawal of some drugs, including alcohol and barbiturates, lowers the seizure threshold in all people [20]. Antidepressants, stimulants, neuroleptics, and sleep preparations all occasionally elicit or allow seizure activity. Amphetamines and tricyclic antidepressants may induce seizure activity as the serum level of the drugs increases [21].

Alcohol

Alcohol withdrawal seizures, also known as *rum fits,* are especially common and can occur after as little as 24 hours of alcohol abuse. Rum fits develop in 4 percent of patients who go on to develop delirium tremens, the acute thought disorder developing in some chronic alcoholics denied alcohol for a few days [20]. The alcohol withdrawal need not be complete for these episodes to occur. Seizures often develop in people who still have relatively high serum alcohol contents. Increasing the risk of seizures in alcoholics and drug abusers is the relatively low seizure threshold that develops with repeated head injuries and poor nutrition (Fig. 4–3) [22].

Seizures associated with alcohol abuse most commonly appear after adolescence [20]. Diagnostic problems arise because the high risk of head trauma in these individuals necessitates investigations for cerebral contusions, subdural hematomas, and posttraumatic meningitis even if the patient has rum fits several times yearly. Increasing the likelihood of intracranial bleeding and infections in these patients are the alcoholic liver damage and other systemic effects that interfere with the production of normal clotting factors and maintenance of an effective immune system.

Therapeutic difficulties also arise because of the behavioral and biochemical characteristics of the chronic alcoholic. These individuals' compliance when they are not intoxicated is erratic, and they can provide no cooperation with a drug regimen when they are intoxicated. Even if they are given the medication regularly by a friend or relative willing to supervise this activity, the metabolism and excretion of the antiepileptic drugs is altered by the chronic ingestion of alcohol [22]. Phenytoin, for example, is turned over more quickly in an alcoholic without terminal liver damage than in a normal person or in an alcoholic with advanced cirrhosis [20].

The risk of status epilepticus faced by all patients with epilepsy is not exaggerated in the alcoholic [20]. This is unexpected, since status epilepticus often occurs with drug withdrawal. Patients developing epilepsy with alcohol abuse may have either generalized or partial seizures. The alcohol withdrawal seizure is usually a generalized tonic-clonic seizure.

Depressants

Barbiturate withdrawal after protracted abuse may be life-threatening [23]. Within 24 hours of stopping the drug, the patient becomes tremulous, restless,

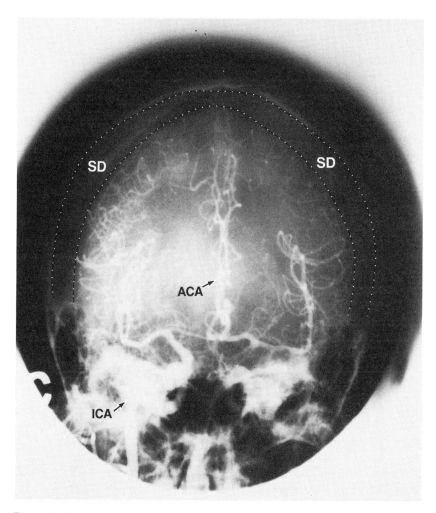

Figure 4–3.
This chronic alcoholic suffered repeated falls that led to these near-lethal bilateral chronic subdural hematomas (SD). The symmetry of the subdural lesions prevented lateral displacement of the anterior cerebral arteries (ACA). The internal carotid artery (ICA) can be seen from its point of entry into the skull.

weak, and febrile. Delirium, sleeplessness, and seizures may develop within 2 or 3 days, and status epilepticus is not an uncommon complication [23]. Similar withdrawal symptoms may develop after protracted methaqualone (Quaālude) abuse, but patients taking this drug in excess may also develop seizures when the drug reaches toxic levels [23]. Withdrawal seizures are best treated with intramuscular phenobarbital (see Chapter 13).

Stimulants

High doses of amphetamines or cocaine can precipitate seizures, but what levels are actually required to cause trouble is unknown. Most reports on the complications of illicit drugs have not been very objective [24]. Part of the inconsistency in experience with these drugs is caused by the uncertain nature of drugs taken illicitly. Cocaine often is adulterated with lidocaine hydrochloride or procaine hydrochloride, because the local anesthetic effects of these drugs imitate the sensation induced by the cocaine when it is inhaled. Amphetamines may also be mixed with the drug to increase the stimulant effect [21]. The patient does not know what he bought, and the physician cannot depend on the drug user's analysis of the material to document which drug is responsible for an adverse reaction.

Precautions

Studies on illicit drugs make it very clear that people with epilepsy should be advised against using any of these drugs for recreation. Marijuana has had no apparent provocative or protective influence on epilepsy, but even this widely used material is commonly adulterated [25]. If the drug use is because of addiction rather than preference, then the patient's addiction must be dealt with at the same time that the epilepsy is managed [24]. Patients who must take antidepressants and who have a low seizure threshold should be managed cautiously because of the tendency of these drugs to lower the seizure threshold still further (see Chapter 12).

Special problems arise with drug abuse in women who are of childbearing age or pregnant. Although seizures may not develop in a pregnant woman addicted to heroin or abusing barbiturates, withdrawal from these drugs can provoke seizures in her newborn infant (see Chapter 5). Anticonvulsants may be needed during the newborn period for a child born to an addicted mother. The addiction will pose many other problems for the newborn, and so such cases should be managed by a neonatologist familiar with the metabolic and neurologic problems that can arise soon after birth.

CAUSES OF EPILEPSY

Although seizures are caused by a wide variety of injuries, infections, and other types of central nervous system insult, not all provocative stimuli will lead to epilepsy. The patient who experiences seizures during meningoencephalitis that disappear with treatment of the infection cannot properly be considered a victim of epilepsy unless a persistent tendency to have seizures is demonstrated by subsequent attacks. Even the alcoholic who has recurrent seizures over the course of years does not have epilepsy if the seizures only occur with alcohol withdrawal. In the final analysis, the vast majority of patients with epilepsy have the disorder as a result of head trauma, inheritance of a nervous system disorder, or for no apparent reason.

REFERENCES

1. Hauser, W.A., Anderson, V.E., Loewenson, R.B., et al. Seizure recurrence after a first unprovoked seizure. *N. Engl. J. Med.* 347(9):522–528, 1982.
2. Booker, H.E. Management of the difficult patient with complex partial seizures. *Adv. Neurol.* 11:369, 1975.
3. DeJong, R.N. *The Neurologic Examination.* New York: Harper & Row, 1979.
4. Meencke, H.J., Janz, D. Neuropathological findings in primary generalized epilepsy: a study of eight cases. *Epilepsia* 25(1):8–21, 1984.
5. Jennett, B., van de Sande, J. EEG prediction of post-traumatic epilepsy. *Epilepsia* 16:251–256, 1975.
6. Jennett, B. Epilepsy after head injury and craniotomy. In Godwin-Austen, R.B., Espir, M.L.E. (eds.), *Driving and Epilepsy.* Royal Society of Medicine International Congress and Symposium Series, no. 60. London: Academic Press, 1983, pp. 49–51.
7. Lechtenberg, R., Vaida, G.A. Schistosomiasis of the spinal cord. *Neurology* (N.Y.) 27:55–59, 1977.
8. Adams, R.D., Victor, M. *Principles of Neurology.* New York: McGraw-Hill Book Co., 1977.
9. Gilman, S., Bloedel, J., Lechtenberg, R. *Disorders of the Cerebellum.* Philadelphia: F.A. Davis Co., 1981.
10. Amici, R., Avanzini, G., Pacini, L. Cerebellar tumors. (Monographs in Neural Sciences. Vol. IV.) Basel, Switzerland: Karger, 1976.
11. Wolf, P. A., Dawber, T.R., Thomas, H.E.J., Kannel, W.B. Epidemiological assessment of chronic atrial fibrillation and stroke: the Framingham study. *Neurology* (N.Y.) 28:973–977, 1978.
12. Meyer, J.S., Charney, J.Z., Rivera, V.M., Mathew, N.T. Cerebral embolization: prospective clinical analysis of 42 cases. *Stroke* 2:541–554, 1971.
13. Ueda, K., Toole, J.F., McHenry, L.C., Jr. Carotid and vertebrobasilar transient ischemic attacks: clinical and angiographic correlation. *Neurology* (N.Y.) 29:1094–1101, 1979.
14. Drake, C.G. Arteriovenous malformations of the brain. *N. Engl. J. Med.* 309(5):308–309, 1983.
15. Bennett, R., Hughes, G.R.V., Bywaters, E.G.L., et al. Neuropsychiatric problems in systemic lupus erythematosus. *Br. Med. J.* 4:342, 1972.
16. Fox, I.S., Spence, A.M., Wheelis, R.F., Healey, L.A. Cerebral embolism in Libman-Sacks endocarditis. *Neurology* (N.Y.) 30:487–491, 1980.
17. Karpati, G., Frame, B. Neuropsychiatric disorders in primary hyperparathyroidism. *Arch. Neurol.* 10:387, 1964.
18. Rosenberg,, R.N. Biochemical genetics of neurologic disease. *N. Engl. J. Med.* 305(20):1181–1193, 1981.
19. DeLong, G.R. Case records of the Massachusetts General Hospital. Case 5, 1982. *N. Engl. J. Med.* 306:286–293, 1982.
20. Hillbom, M.E. Occurrence of cerebral seizures provoked by alcohol abuse. *Epilepsia* 21:459–466, 1980.

21. Angrist, B.M.   Toxic manifestations of amphetamine. *Psychiatr. Ann.* 8:443, 1978.
22. Mendelson, J.H., Mellow, N.K.   Biologic concomitants of alcoholism. *N. Engl. J. Med.* 301:912, 1979.
23. Drugs of choice. New Rochelle, N.Y.: The Medical Letter, 1977, pp. 45–63.
24. Pope, H.G.   Drug abuse and psychopathology. *N. Engl. J. Med.* 301:1341, 1979.
25. Relman, A.S.   Marijuana and health. *N. Engl. J. Med.* 306(10):603–605, 1982.

5. Causes of Epilepsy in Infancy and Childhood

Some types of epilepsy and problems that cause epilepsy only develop, or are much more likely to develop, during infancy or childhood rather than in adult life. This is not simply because the infant or young child exhibits perinatal problems that become less acute as the child ages, but also because the infant's brain is different from the child's brain, just as the child's brain is different from the adult's. Each is vulnerable to its own spectrum of problems and each responds somewhat differently to the same stimuli.

Some problems, such as perinatal infections and developmental defects that limit the infants viability, can occur only in infancy or childhood. Perinatal hypoxia or subarachnoid hemorrhage often produce seizures during the first few days of life as well as later in life. Congenital brain malformations can lead to seizures that first appear when an individual is 30 or 40 years old, but they are more likely to be symptomatic in infancy or childhood. Hereditary metabolic problems, in which seizure disorders are an early manifestation, also are much more likely to become symptomatic in childhood than in adult life, whereas brain tumors are less likely to be the cause of seizures in children than in adults. Accidental poisoning is a minor cause of epilepsy in adults but a major cause in children.

Head trauma causes brain damage and seizures at all ages, but it is a particularly common cause of seizures in young children [1]. In fact, head trauma is the commonest identifiable cause of nonfebrile seizures in children younger than 7 years. It accounts for approximately 34 percent of the nonfebrile seizures in this group [1]. The risks associated with head trauma vary with the age of the child and the maturity of his nervous system, but at any age, an adequately violent blow to the head can initiate seizure activity.

Epilepsy in children may develop within minutes of birth or late in adolescence. The age at which seizures appear often is related to the type of epilepsy that develops or to the lesion causing the seizures. Certain patterns of epilepsy, such as salaam attacks and infantile spasms, invariably appear in infancy, and others, such as benign juvenile myoclonic epilepsy, are more typical of adolescence.

If a metabolic problem is responsible for the seizures, the age of seizure onset reflects the pace at which the metabolic disease disrupts the normal brain activity. Seizure may appear within the first few months of life in individuals with Tay-Sachs disease and may not appear until adolescence in others with neuronal ceroid lipofuscinosis, even though both of these rare nervous system diseases involve the abnormal accumulation of materials in neurons of the cerebral cortex.

SEIZURES IN THE NEWBORN

Seizures are the most common neurologic problem in newborn infants [2]. Approximately 0.8 percent of neonates have seizures [3]. The newborn period is defined as the first 28 days of life, but much of the seizure activity observed in neonates will occur in the first 3 days of life [1]. Although relatively few newborns have seizures, the fraction of critically ill neonates who have seizures is substantial (up to 20 percent of the infants in neonatal intensive care units) [3]. Of all the children who have seizures by the time they are 7 years old, approximately 10 percent have neonatal seizures [1]. The incidence of seizures unrelated to fever during infancy and childhood is highest in the first month of life [1].

When neonatal seizures develop, they usually occur in rapid succession over several hours or days [2]. Twenty percent of infants who have neonatal

Table 5-1.
Percentage of Children Who Exhibit Their First Seizure Before 7 Years of Age

Age (years)	Generalized Seizures (%)	Minor Motor Seizures (%)	Focal Motor Seizures (%)	Absence Seizures (%)	All Seizure Types (%)
0.1–0.5	23.1	42.0	20.4	0.0	22.2
>0.5–1.0	8.5	16.0	7.5	7.7	8.8
>1–2	16.1	8.0	12.9	15.4	14.8
>2–3	15.8	10.0	12.9	11.5	14.0
>3–4	11.1	16.0	17.2	15.4	13.3
>4–7	25.3	8.0	29.0	50.0	26.9

Table 5–2.
Causes of Neonatal Seizures

Asphyxia	Transient metabolic disorders:
Intracranial hemorrhage, idiopathic or	hypocalcemia, hypoglycemia,
traumatic	hypomagnesemia, hyponatremia,
Intrauterine or perinatal infection	hypernatremia
Congenital brain malformation	Inborn errors of metabolism
Drug withdrawal (with an addicted	Familial CNS disorders
mother)	Pyridoxine deficiency
Local anesthetic intoxication	Idiopathic epilepsy

seizures for whatever reason will have seizures unrelated to fevers later in childhood (Table 5–1) [1]. Two-thirds of these subsequent seizures occur by 6 months of age; three-fourths occur by 1 year. The child at highest risk for subsequent epilepsy is the one with obvious structural brain damage, whereas the one at lowest risk has a correctable metabolic disorder.

A fairly limited range of problems can cause seizures during the newborn period [4]. Common etiologies are asphyxia, intracranial hemorrhage, and nervous system infections (Table 5–2) [3]. In many cases, no etiology will be apparent until months or years after the appearance of the seizures.

The commonest seizure types during the newborn period and the first year of life include minor motor seizures and infantile spasms. The patterns of seizures observed in the neonate are not at all like those that develop as the child gets older, at least partly because the brain at the time of birth has not reached the level of organization typical of the older child [5]. Most of the seizures occurring during the first few days and weeks of life are fairly subtle (and are classified as such), often consisting of little more than paroxysmal deviation of the eyes or repetitive blinking [2]. More obvious tonic or clonic seizures are less common than the subtle seizures, but they, too, do not resemble childhood or even later infantile generalized seizures [5]. Infantile spasms with massive myoclonic jerks may be more apparent as the child leaves the newborn period. Sixty percent of the children who ever develop minor motor seizures or infantile spasms do so by 1 year of age [1].

Hypoxic or Ischemic Brain Damage

Approximately 65 percent of neonatal seizures are caused by hypoxic or ischemic brain damage [5, 6]. Seizures caused by this inadequate delivery of oxygen to the brain usually appear within the first 24 hours of life. Most of these children have suffered asphyxia while still in the uterus rather than during or after delivery [5]. Inadequate oxygenation or blood flow to the fetal brain may occur for many reasons, including problems in the placenta (e.g., premature separation from the wall of the uterus), problems in the fetal circulatory system (e.g., heart or vascular anomalies), or hematologic catastrophes (e.g., Rh incompatibility).

Any child with early-onset seizures must be investigated for causes of seizure activity other than asphyxia, simply because many of these children also exhibit hypoglycemia and hypocalcemia. Asphyxia may inaccurately be presumed to be the cause of seizures in any child who has problems breathing at birth or who is delivered with the umbilical cord tightly bound about its neck. However, problems with breathing may be a result, rather than the cause, of brain damage. Caution is especially appropriate in evaluating premature infants, who may have intraventricular hemorrhages that cause, rather than result from, respiratory problems.

Injuries to the brain at birth are loosely included in the group of perinatal injuries called *cerebral palsy*. Epilepsy does not always develop with this type of brain injury, but it may appear years after all other neurologic problems caused by the birth injury have stabilized. Cerebral palsy is, by definition, a static encephalopathy—that is, a problem in the brain that will not cause progressive damage after the initial insult—but the appearance of epilepsy as a symptom of this condition may be delayed for months or years.

Asphyxia is obviously not limited to the prenatal or perinatal period and may occur during childhood with drowning or strangulation. Weeks or months after a drowning accident, the child may develop intellectual, affective, or seizure disorders that are not apparent immediately after the child regains consciousness [7]. When seizures occur with this type of hypoxic injury, long-term antiepileptic treatment usually is needed.

Intracranial Hemorrhage

Subarachnoid, intraventricular, and intracerebral hemorrhages all can cause seizures in the neonatal period. Subarachnoid hemorrhages not secondary to trauma usually become evident on the second day of life and are three times as common in premature infants as they are in full-term infants [5]. Intraventricular hemorrhages during the newborn period occur almost exclusively in premature infants. They appear because of the instability of the blood vessels in the premature infant's brain. With substantial perinatal trauma, the infant may develop contusions in the brain, occasionally associated with subdural hematomas [5]. If these contusions are going to induce seizure activity, they usually will do so within the first 24 hours of life.

Intrauterine and Perinatal Infection

In some instances, an infection acquired before or at the time of birth causes brain damage that is later manifested as slow intellectual development, poor gait, impaired hearing, or other neurologic deficits. Intrauterine infections with a variety of agents, including coxsackie B virus, *Herpes simplex,* rubella, toxoplasmosis, and cytomegalovirus, may leave the infant with brain damage that leads to epilepsy in the neonatal period or years after birth. Twelve percent of neonatal seizures are caused by central nervous system infections [5]. If the child is born prematurely, the most likely responsible bacterial agent is *Escherichia coli*. If the neonate is a full-term infant, the most likely bacterium is a group B beta-hemolytic streptococcus [5].

Calcifications in the brain, chorioretinitis, and other signs of nervous system damage usually appear along with the seizure activity if the intrauterine infection involved toxoplasmosis or cytomegalovirus. Some infections are picked up at the time of delivery rather than while the fetus is developing in the uterus. Exposure to *Herpes simplex* type 2 in the birth canal may cause an encephalitis that leaves the infant with mental retardation and a low seizure threshold. The risk of central nervous system injury from such a virus is substantial enough that cesarean section often is performed when this type of herpetic infection is evident in or near the mother's vagina.

Metabolic Problems

The most easily managed neonatal seizures are those due to reversible metabolic abnormalities, such as hypoglycemia, hypocalcemia, and hypomagnesemia. More complex metabolic problems from inborn errors of metabolism usually are untreatable, and so the delays invariably assoicated with confirming the diagnosis of a lipidosis or amino acid disturbance generally are unimportant from the point of view of the newborn's welfare. However, there are notable exceptions, such as phenylketonuria. Therefore, neonatal screening tests for metabolic disorders should be done as rapidly and accurately as possible whenever there is reason to suspect a metabolic problem.

Hypoglycemia
Hypoglycemia can cause neonatal seizures, but it commonly occurs with neonatal seizures that result from several other disturbances. A diagnosis of hypoglycemia in a child does not exclude the possibility of meningitis, hypocalcemia, or subarachnoid hemorrhage. Children most likely to develop hypoglycemia sufficient to trigger neonatal seizures are those born to diabetic mothers and those with very low birth weights [5]. Seizures from hypoglycemia usually start on the second day of life and may respond dramatically to intravenous dextrose without any other antiepileptic treatment. At what level of serum glucose the child should be considered hypoglycemic is controversial, but neonatologists generally agree that a blood glucose level of less than 30 mg/dl in the full-term infant or 20 mg/dl in the premature infant is dangerously low [5]. When hypoglycemia is found, the possible coincidence of other disturbances of blood chemistries should still be assessed.

Hypocalcemia and Hypomagnesemia
Hypocalcemia in the newborn is defined as a serum calcium content of less than 7 mg/dl [5]. Infants with obvious hypocalcemia may be having seizures induced by other metabolic problems, and so investigation of the infant should

not stop with the identification of a low serum calcium content. Magnesium and calcium metabolism are closely linked, and both must be evaluated when either appears to be abnormal.

Infants developing seizures strictly on the basis of hypocalcemia usually do so by the fourth day of life. The neonates at high risk for hypocalcemia are those with low birth weights and those who suffered substantial trauma at the time of delivery [5]. Apparently, an inadequate endocrine response to the stress induced by the injuries, rather than the actual binding of calcium in injured organs, is responsible for this hypocalcemia. The child with a normal birth weight who develops seizures on the sixth or seventh day after birth is likely to be hypomagnesemic, which is the basis for the seizures, even if hypocalcemia is found. Disturbed parathyroid gland function plays a large role in many of these neonatal calcium disturbances.

Other Electrolyte Disturbances

Phosphorus levels are routinely elevated when calcium levels are low. The extent to which this contributes to neonatal seizures is unknown. Serum sodium may be low enough during the neonatal period to induce seizures, but hyponatremia in this stage of infancy usually is from inappropriate antidiuretic hormone production associated with a meningitis [5]. Hypernatremia sometimes induces neonatal seizure activity, but this generally develops only with severe dehydration.

In some infants and children, congenital renal disease, either by interfering with the maintenance of sodium, potassium, or calcium levels or by leading to uremia, may lower the seizure threshold adequately to provoke seizures. Seizure activity in this context is more appropriately regarded as a sign of metabolic encephalopathy than epilepsy. Although these seizures may recur, the treatment required to suppress them is correction of the metabolic problem. Antiepileptic drugs may be needed while other measures, such as dialysis, are employed to correct the metabolic defect, but chronic antiepileptic medication usually is unnecessary.

Inborn Errors of Metabolism

Defects in the metabolism of several different substances can lead to neonatal seizures. The system at fault may be required to metabolize lipids, carbohydrates, or amino acids. Many of these disorders are inherited in autosomal recessive patterns, and so there may be little to indicate that the child will develop problems until the first neonatal seizure occurs.

During the neonatal period, the commonest disturbance of amino acid metabolism likely to precipitate seizures is maple syrup urine disease [8]. This is a disorder of branched-chain amino acid (leucine, isoleucine, valine) metabolism [9]. By 24 hours after birth, most infants with this disorder will have markedly elevated plasma leucine levels and a metabolic acidosis [9]. The distinctive smell and appearance of the urine simplifies the diagnosis of maple syrup urine disease, but there is still no effective way to treat this inborn error of metabolism.

A more manageable disturbance of amino acid metabolism is phenylketonuria. It is less likely than maple syrup urine disease to cause seizures in the newborn period, but it can be detected by 24 hours after birth and managed with dietary precautions [10]. Phenylalanine must be excluded from the diet, but even with rigorous efforts to limit the intake of this amino acid, the child may develop dementia [8].

Some children have an excessive need for pyridoxine and have neonatal seizures when routine intake of pyridoxine is not supplemented. The simplest way to identify this disorder is by conducting a therapeutic trial with pyridoxine while the newborn is having a seizure [5]. In a positive test, the seizure usually will stop and the child's electroencephalogram will become more normal as the excess pyridoxine is infused.

Inborn errors of metabolism that cause deranged metabolic activity at the level of the neuron (diseases such as Tay-Sachs disease and neuronal ceroid lipofuscinosis) precipitate seizures as metabolic waste products accumulate in the gray matter of the brain [8]. Seizures develop in childhood in most affected individuals, but they may not be evident until long after the newborn period.

Excessively high levels of bilirubin in the neonate, whether from hepatic problems or hemolysis, can damage the brain as part of the disturbance called *kernicterus*. Hyperbilirubinemia is actually a relatively rare cause of seizures in the newborn period, but half of all infants with kernicterus will develop seizures [5]. The profound jaundice evident in the infant simplifies the diagnosis. Structural damage occurring with kernicterus can be minimized with aggressive treatment of the hyperbilirubinemia.

Developmental Defects

Neonatal seizures may also appear because of developmental abnormalities in the central nervous system. Systemic signs may provide some clue to the nature of the brain abnormality. A large facial port-wine spot may occur with Sturge-Weber syndrome, a developmental abnormality causing brain damage and vascular abnormalities with associated seizure disorders. With neurofibromatosis (von Recklinghausen disease) and tuberous sclerosis, gross structural abnormalities in the brain and hyperpigmented or hypopigmented spots in the skin may be associated with various types of epilepsies that appear during the first few months or years of life. Von Hippel-Lindau disease may present with renal, ovarian, or liver masses and is associated with hemangiomas in the nervous system that induce seizures when they bleed. Any child with seizures must be carefully examined for these and other clues to the central nervous system disease responsible for the seizures.

Drug Withdrawal

If the infant's mother has abused an addicting drug at about the time of the delivery, the newborn is likely to go through drug withdrawal. With narcotic withdrawal, neonatal seizures are fairly unlikely, although they certainly do occur [5]. The addicted mother whose child is at greatest risk is the one who abuses short-acting barbiturates, such as secobarbital sodium (Seconal). Withdrawal seizures with any of these medications usually occur during the first 2 or 3 days of life. Most infants exhibiting symptoms of narcotic withdrawal have a high-pitched cry, hypertonia, sneezing, vomiting, and jitteriness rather than true seizures [5]. Infants suffering any type of drug withdrawal are also at high risk for hypoglycemia and so several factors may actually precipitate the neonatal seizure.

An infant delivered by a mother who has had a local anesthetic injection to produce a cervical block occasionally will develop withdrawal seizures. These occur if the child is inadvertently injected with the short-acting anesthetic. This complication has been most often described after mepivacaine hydrochloride injections [5].

INFANTILE SPASMS

Infantile spasms are a diverse group of generalized seizures caused by the same problems that can produce neonatal seizures. What is distinctive about them is that they usually appear at approximately the third to seventh month of life, are often associated with diffusely disorganized electroencephalographic patterns called *hypsarrhythmias,* and involve prominent muscle spasms or jerking movements. Of the cases of infantile spasm that have an obvious etiology, approximately 35 percent are secondary to asphyxia [11]. Central nervous system developmental problems are also a common cause of these seizures, and the most common dysgenesis associated with infantile spasms is that caused by tuberous sclerosis, a dominantly inherited disorder of nervous system development with variable penetrance. Approximately 39 percent of infantile spasms are idiopathic [11]. Male infants are affected almost twice as often as females.

During the attacks, the child usually has a brief spasm that causes an apparent limb jerk. These spasms generally occur in clusters and are triggered by arousal from sleep or drowsiness [12]. The infant often cries at the end of a cluster of spasms.

Approximately 25 percent of the children who have infantile spasms die, most by the age of 3 years [12]. In those who survive, the infantile spasms invariably stop by 5 years of age. However, at least half of the children who exhibit this disorder will continue to have seizures, and 77 percent are obviously mentally retarded [11, 12]. The seizures developing after infantile spasms usually are generalized tonic-clonic, but some are focal or atonic. Early and aggressive treatment is appropriate (see Chapter 13).

FEBRILE SEIZURES

Seizures occurring when a child develops a high fever are called *febrile seizures* or *febrile convulsions.* These usually are generalized seizures with tonic-clonic limb movements and loss of consciousness. Between birth and 5 years of age, approximately 2 percent of all infants will have febrile seizures and an additional 1 percent will have seizures unrelated to fever [13]. If a child has a neurologic injury, infection, or malformation, he is very likely to have a febrile seizure during his first year of life [1].

Nearly 75 percent of all seizures occurring before 7 years of age are associated with a fever [1]. Half of all children who develop symptomatic seizures with a fever do so by 1 year of age. Most symptomatic febrile seizures are from central nervous system infections; 62 percent are from meningitis or encephalitis [1].

Febrile illness may also precipitate seizures by producing metabolic problems, such as those that develop with diarrheal diseases. Homeostatic mechanisms may be unable to keep pace with the loss of electrolytes into the stool. Hypokalemia or hypomagnesemia may develop. Dehydration from fluid loss may produce hypernatremia as well.

The interval between a febrile seizure and subsequent nonfebrile seizures may be very long, averaging 23 months for those patients who develop nonfebrile seizures after having a febrile seizure [1]. Most children with febrile seizures never have a nonfebrile seizure.

Simple and Complex Febrile Seizures

If the seizure occurs when the child is between 1 and 5 years of age, is nonfocal, lasts less than 15 minutes, and is unassociated with any persistent neurologic deficits, and if no other family member has epilepsy, it is called a *simple febrile seizure* (Table 5–3) [14]. Distinguishing this simple seizure from the *complex febrile seizure,* which lasts more than 15 minutes, has focal features and persistent neurologic signs, occurs before 1 year of age, or is associated with a family history of nonfebrile seizures, is important for deciding on therapy [14]. Simple febrile seizures need not be managed with antiepileptic drugs, whereas the complex type must be. The simple seizures are best treated with antipyretics, an alcohol rub, baths, and the like. In the complex form, the underlying problem, if evident, must be managed.

Children with complex febrile seizures develop nonfebrile seizures in 10 percent of cases, whereas those with simple febrile seizures have nonfebrile episodes in only 2.2 percent of cases [14]. Fortunately, at least 2 of 3 children

Table 5–3.
Febrile Seizures

Simple	Complex
Onset at 1–5 years old	Onset before 1 year of age
Generalized	Partial—simple or complex
Less than 15 minutes long	More than 15 minutes long
No other affected family members	Associated with history of seizures in family members
No apparent brain damage	Persistent neurologic signs

Treatment

Antipyretics, alcohol rub, baths, etc.	Antiepileptics
	Management of underlying problem if evident

with febrile seizures have simple febrile seizures. One of 3 children who have had a simple febrile seizure will, at some time, have a second seizure of the same type [14]. Obviously, the children most likely to have nonfebrile seizures after a febrile one are those with discrete neurologic deficits. Any child who has developmental delays or focal neurologic deficits and a febrile seizure should be started on antiepileptic therapy after the first seizure.

Status epilepticus may occur with febrile seizures, and when it does, it often accompanies the first febrile seizure [14]. This is a dangerous but treatable problem, which requires intensive monitoring of the child until seizures have stopped for at least 24 hours.

Familial Patterns

Febrile seizures do exhibit familial patterns of incidence. Children with more than three episodes of febrile seizures have relatives with febrile seizures in three of five cases [15]. This simply indicates that the child and other affected family members share low seizure thresholds: Relatively minor stimuli, such as high fevers, are enough to elicit a full-blown seizure in these related individuals. If a child has febrile seizures, the likelihood that its sibling will also have febrile seizures is approximately 10 to 15 percent [16]. This concordance is even greater when the sibling is the identical twin of the individual with febrile seizures [16]. Infants with similar genetic compositions and intrauterine experiences have similar susceptibilities to febrile seizures.

Investigations

Any child who has a febrile seizure for the first time should be hospitalized for observation and evaluation. In children younger than 3 years, the risk of meningitis is substantial and the signs of infection can be very subtle [14]. It is unarguably wise to err on the side of caution and perform a lumbar puncture (spinal tap) to check the cerebrospinal fluid for infection. This is especially urgent for infants younger than 6 months, in whom a bacterial meningitis may present with little more than fever and a febrile seizure. Failure to detect a meningitis or meningoencephalitis early in its evolution may mean permanent retardation or death for the affected infant.

Febrile seizures rarely occur in children older than 7 years [15]. The fever cannot be assumed to be a major factor in the genesis of seizures occurring after 5 years of age. These prepubertal children should be investigated for vascular malformations, subarachnoid hemorrhages, tumors, and central nervous system infections.

Although the electroencephalogram is abnormal in 2 of 3 children with febrile seizures, the abnormal pattern does not necessarily help distinguish simple from complex seizures [15]. Some physicians believe that a febrile seizure associated with a focal or paroxysmal abnormality on the electroencephalogram must be considered complex. The value of this rule is controversial, but it certainly aids in decision making on treatment in ambiguous cases. The child with a focal or paroxysmal pattern should be given antiepileptic medications (see Chapter 13).

POISONING

Poisoning accounts for approximately 20 percent of the symptomatic non-febrile seizures that occur in children younger than 7 years [1]. This high incidence of toxic encephalopathy reflects the early childhood practice of ingesting all types of materials. The toxic substance may be medication intended for an adult: Overdoses of aspirin and sleep medications are fairly common, although these usually do not cause seizures. Antiepileptic drugs are not necessary in cases of such poisoning, unless recurrent seizures develop while the poison is being eliminated from the child's body. If the child ingests an overdose of a barbiturate, the seizure activity may not become apparent until the level of barbiturate in the blood falls substantially.

The one poison to which children have special access and susceptibility is lead [1]. They often ingest lead from soil, paint, plaster, and other materials that adults rarely swallow [17, 18]. Lead encephalopathy usually causes generalized tonic-clonic (grand mal) convulsions. Permanent brain damage from this heavy metal poison may necessitate long-term antiepileptic treatment to suppress seizures.

With every poison, the most important goal is to minimize the damage done by the toxic substance. Rapid clearance of the poison and close observation of the child during the time it takes to eliminate it is essential. If seizures complicate the poisoning, antiepileptics may be required for days or weeks after the incident.

IMPLICATIONS

The types of problems that cause seizures in infancy and childhood generally demand urgent attention. It is true that the adult with meningitis also needs rapid assessment and treatment, but delays in diagnosis and treatment in infants and children more often have dire consequences. The bases for most neonatal seizures will kill or severely impair the infant unless appropriate corrective steps are taken within hours or days. The disorders in which truly corrective treatment is not an option, such as intrauterine infections and intraventricular hemorrhages, present enormous management problems [19]. The child with ischemic brain damage may need antiepileptic therapy as well as physical therapy to maximize its independence. Early recognition of the cause of the seizures in infants and children gives the affected child the best chance for survival and maximizing its abilities.

REFERENCES

1. Ellenberg, J.H., Hirtz, D.G., Nelson, K.B. Age at onset of seizures in young children. *Ann. Neurol.* 15(2):127–134, 1984.
2. Aicardi, J. Neonatal and infantile seizures. In Morselli, P.L., Pippenger, C.E., Penry, J.K. (eds.), *Antiepileptic Drug Therapy in Pediatrics.* New York: Raven Press, 1983, pp. 103–113.
3. Gal, P., Toback, J., Boer, H.R., et al. Efficacy of phenobarbital monotherapy in treatment of neonatal seizures—relationship to blood levels. *Neurology* (N.Y.) 32(12):1401–1404, 1982.
4. Lombroso, C.T. Differentiation of seizures in newborns and in early infancy. In Morselli, P.L., Pippenger, C.E., Penry, J.K. (eds.), *Antiepileptic Drug Therapy in Pediatrics.* New York: Raven Press, 1983, pp. 85–102.
5. Volpe, J.J. Neonatal seizures. *Clin. Perinatol.* 4(1):43–63, 1977.
6. Hauser, W.A., Anderson, V.E., Loewenson, R.B., et al. Seizure recurrence after a first unprovoked seizure. *N. Engl. J. Med.* 307(9):522–528, 1982.
7. Lechtenberg, R. *The Psychiatrist's Guide to Diseases of the Nervous System.* New York: John Wiley & Sons, 1982.
8. Rosenberg, R.N. Biochemical genetics of neurologic disease. *N. Engl. J. Med.* 305(20):1181–1193, 1981.
9. DiGeorge, A.M., Rezvani, I., Garibaldi, L.R., Schwartz, M. Prospective study of maple-syrup-urine disease for the first four days of life. *N. Engl. J. Med.* 307:1492–1495, 1982.
10. Schneider, A.J. Newborn phenylalanine/tyrosine metabolism: implictions for screening for phenylketonuria. *Am. J. Dis. Child.* 137:427–432, 1983.
11. Lombroso, C.T. A prospective study of infantile spasms: clinical and therapeutic correlations. *Epilepsia* 24(2):135–158, 1983.
12. Friedman, E., Pampiglione, G. Prognostic implications of electroencephalographic findings of hypsarrhythmia in first year of life. *Br. Med. J.* 4:323–325, 1971.
13. Berg, B.O. Prognosis of childhood epilepsy—another look. *N. Engl. J. Med.* 306(14):861–862, 1982.
14. Febrile convulsions. *Br. Med. J.* 282(6265):673–674, 1981.
15. Goodey, R.J. Drugs in the treatment of tinnitus. *Ciba Found. Symp.* 85:263–278, 1981.

16. Jennings, M.T., Bird, T.D.   Genetic influences in the epilepsies. *Am. J. Dis. Child.* 135:450–457, 1981.
17. Mahaffey, K.R., Annest, J.L., Roberts, J., et al.   National estimates of blood levels: United States, 1976–1980. *N. Engl. J. Med.* 307(10):573–579, 1982.
18. Lin-Fu, J.S.   Children and lead. New findings and concerns. *N. Engl. J. Med.* 307(10):615–616, 1982.
19. Rapin, I.   *Children with Brain Dysfunction. Neurology, Cognition, Language, and Behavior.* New York: Raven Press, 1982, p. 284.

6. Investigation of the Patient with Epilepsy

Once epilepsy is suspected, a systematic investigation of the patient will determine if epilepsy is responsible for the behavior arousing concern and if the abnormal signs and symptoms are caused by a treatable lesion. Every investigation must include a thorough consideration of the patient's work and home life, habits, and addictions. Systemic problems should not be overlooked, and hereditary problems must be considered. The diagnostic procedures needed to investigate the patient will be determined by the diagnoses that the history and physical examination suggest.

The age of the patient when epilepsy is first suspected plays a major role in deciding what tests are appropriate for evaluating that patient. A girl whose seizures start when she is 10 years of age will be subjected to fewer and less invasive tests than a woman whose seizures begin at 40. The young person probably has idiopathic seizures if no other neurologic problems are evident on a routine examination, whereas the adult is at high risk for a brain tumor or central nervous system infection, even if the neurologic examination is normal. Discrimination is important in choosing the techniques to be used, not simply because many of the tests are expensive and time consuming, but also because some of them provide little information that will be useful in reaching a diagnosis or deciding on therapy. Some diagnostic techniques currently used for the investigation of neurologic problems are experimental and, though they may one day be very important in the routine evaluation of people with epilepsy, their usefulness in this arena remains to be established.

The least expensive and most informative part of any evaluation is the patient history and physical examination.

HISTORY

Every evaluation of any patient with episodes of altered consciousness, transient involuntary movements, or fleeting sensory phenomena must include questions that optimally clarify what the patient has been experiencing [1, 2]. A poor history often is responsible for delays in recognizing seizures as the cause of altered consciousness or abnormal movements [2]. In most illnesses, the patient can provide enough details about the problem to direct further investigations, but with epilepsy, the history must often be obtained from family, friends, and co-workers who witness the patient's worrisome episodes. The patient rarely can provide an adequate description of what happened during or before the episode. In fact, many patients who experience seizures are unaware that anything at all occurs and often resent the urging of family and friends that they consult a physician [3]. Events following the episode frequently are remembered in a fragmented way, and numerous irrelevant activities that preceded the episode will be unduly emphasized. Most patients want to forget the episode and so will ascribe it to a transient problem, such as an argument, a bad meal, or a change in the weather.

Health professionals familiar with epilepsy are the best observers, but they rarely witness the initial seizures. Because there are usually no truly perceptive observers present during the episode arousing concern, the patient and those witnessing the attack must be questioned about specific features of the episode. Events preceding any obvious change in consciousness or behavior, anything that occurred during the period of altered consciousness, and the personality changes, disorientation, or weakness that were present after the acute episode must be characterized in detail [4]. Urinary and fecal incontinence must be asked about specifically. The patient should also be questioned about changes in his sleeping pattern and the appearance of enuresis, nocturnal tongue biting, and unexplained nocturnal bruising [5].

Every history must include an extensive past, family, and travel history. Past injuries or illnesses that could lead to seizures should be sought. Head trauma is obviously an important area of concern, but most patients have had what they consider severe head trauma at some time in their lives. The clinician should ask about loss of consciousness, posttraumatic amnesia, and other more objective signs of severe trauma. Patients who describe themselves as moderate or social drinkers should be asked to translate this into an estimate of average weekly alcohol consumption. Few alcoholics recognize their drinking habits as excessive, but alcohol often plays a large role in the development or persistence of seizures.

Remote events may be as important as recent problems. If the patient had

Table 6–1.
Investigation of Neonatal Seizures

Check serum glucose immediately (with Dextrostix reagent strips or similar test)
Check serum calcium, magnesium, bilirubin, and electrolytes
Perform lumbar puncture to look for infection or hemorrhage
Review maternal history for drug abuse, diabetes, etc.
Perform urinalysis, including amino acid studies
Institute trial of pyridoxine
Obtain computed tomogram of head
Obtain interictal electroencephalogram
Perform further biochemical studies using fibroblast cultures and the like if all of the above
    tests are unrevealing

transient alterations of consciousness when he was a child, the likelihood of epilepsy increases. If siblings, parents, or more distant relatives have syncope or seizures, the possibility of a hereditary disorder must be considered. Individuals traveling to areas in which certain diseases associated with epilepsy, such as cysticercosis and schistosomiasis, are endemic should be questioned about dietary and sanitary practices while they were in these regions.

As discussed in Chapter 1, the tendency of many individuals to conceal information complicates the investigation of the patient with epilepsy. The patient may be too embarrassed to report enuresis or fecal incontinence. Even family and friends witnessing the attacks may hesitate to disclose all that they noticed before, during, or after the episodes. For instance, these observers may fail to discuss personality changes that they have noticed in the patient, because they are afraid of offending him.

Inevitably, there are patients for whom little or no history is available. The extreme case of this is the newborn. Although the maternal history may provide some clues about the cause of an infant's seizures, the investigation and management of the patient must proceed based on little more than the history of the pregnancy and delivery. This is especially unfortunate in the newborn because the evaluation of the patient must be done very rapidly and treatment must be instituted as soon as possible (Table 6–1) [6]. The newborn's seizures usually are witnessed by medical personnel, but, at this early age, the pattern of the seizure is so different from childhood or adult seizures that only very perceptive staff can give an adequately detailed description to provide clues to the etiology of the seizures. Even with well-characterized seizures, the possible causes will be multiple, and laboratory investigations, physical examination, and ancillary studies must be relied on heavily.

PHYSICAL EXAMINATION

A comprehensive neurologic examination is only part of the physical examination appropriate for any individual thought to have had a seizure [1].

Attention to systems outside the nervous system often provide clues to the problem inside it. Multiple large café au lait spots on the skin will increase the likelihood that von Recklinghausen disease (neurofibromatosis) is causing the central nervous system disorder. Depigmented spots on the trunk may be associated with tuberous sclerosis; a malar rash, with systemic lupus erythematosus; and a facial port-wine spot, with Sturge-Weber syndrome. Because syncope can imitate seizure activity in older people, the heart must be particularly scrutinized. An arrhythmia apparent only on 24-hour monitoring may be the entire explanation for the transient loss of consciousness thought to be epilepsy. A heart murmur may reflect valvular heart disease that is responsible for emboli to the brain and the resulting transient ischemic attacks.

Even if the probable seizure occurred days or weeks before the patient seeks medical attention, a complete blood count and urinalysis should be performed and blood chemistries should be carefully examined. A persistent electrolyte problem, such as hypocalcemia, may cause intermittent seizures when other disposing factors, such as sleep deprivation, lower the seizure threshold. Liver and kidney function studies may reveal hepatic or renal disease linked to the nervous system problem. A routine electrocardiogram may reveal a heart block that accounts for the syncope.

Even if a nonneurologic basis for the altered consciousness is discovered, a neurologic examination should be conducted. The neurologic examination need not be exhaustive, but the examining physician should be familiar with neurologic problems [2, 7]. A systematic evaluation of speech, mentation, and affect will require some help from individuals familiar with the patient so that recent changes in ability can be appreciated. The evaluation of the cranial nerves, sensory function, motor function, coordination, and reflexes must all take into account medications and procedures to which the patient has been exposed [1].

Skull roentgenograms were a standard part of every neurologic evaluation in the past, but many physicians believe their value is too limited to justify obtaining them for every patient who complains of problems referrable to the head. The lesions most easily seen on routine skull studies, such as an enlarged sella turcica from a pituitary mass or hyperostosis associated with a meningioma, are uncommon in patients with epilepsy except as incidental findings. If the patient has headache or focal signs and epilepsy, more sophisticated radiologic studies, such as computed tomography of the brain or cerebral angiography, will be performed, and skull roentgenograms may provide no additional information. Skull studies are benign and may reveal unexpected problems, but they rarely are helpful in the investigation of seizures.

ELECTROENCEPHALOGRAPHY

Electroencephalography is the study of electrical activity in the brain. The electroencephalograph amplifies and displays voltage changes in only the most superficial layers of the brain, but, despite this limitation, it has been exceedingly useful in the study and characterization of epilepsy. Deflections of its voltage-sensitive needles are recorded by pens on a moving sheet of paper, resulting in the permanent record of brain wave activity, called the *electroencephalogram*. Electrodes are glued to the patient's scalp and ears according to an internationally adopted scheme that maximizes the area of the brain which can be evaluated during a routine study. The machine actually displays the voltage differences between pairs of electrodes. Precisely which pairs of electrodes are used at any one time is determined by settings on the machine.

Electroencephalography has been useful in diagnosing many neurologic problems, but it has made its greatest and most enduring contribution in the investigation of epilepsy. Patients with a structurally normal brain may have seizures, but the electroencephalogram will not be normal in most cases of epilepsy. Although an abnormal electroencephalogram does not indicate that an individual will necessarily have a seizure disorder, it may reinforce one's suspicion of seizure activity in patients with poorly understood motor, sensory, or psychic phenomena [8].

Normal and Abnormal Records

Physicians who have no special interest in interpreting electroencephalograms still are obliged to understand what is said by those who do read electroencephalograms. The technique involves relatively few basic concepts, and, with these in mind, the value and limitations of the procedure can be better appreciated. The electroencephalograph displays brain activity as waves and spikes of varying amplitudes and frequency (Fig. 6–1) [9]. These waves and spikes represent changes in voltage with time over restricted areas of the cortex.

If there is no electrical activity in the cortex, the electroencephalogram will consist of flat lines, a pattern called *isoelectric*. If an abnormal pattern appears over only one side of the head or seems to originate in a restricted part of the cortex, it is called *focal*. Focal spike activity and focal slow wave activity usually indicate brain damage or an irritative lesion (Fig. 6–2). They are the simplest patterns to identify on the electroencephalogram, because of the asymmetry they produce. Spikes are just very brief waves of sufficient amplitude to be distinguished from minor fluctuations in the background. A spike usually lasts less than 80 milliseconds and is very sharply contoured (see Fig. 2–2). If a wave is sharply contoured and lasts more than 80 milliseconds but less than 0.2 seconds, it is called a *sharp wave*.

Several electroencephalographic patterns are normal in children and adults. The most consistent brain wave pattern is alpha activity. This is 8- to 12-Hz waveforms evident over at least the occipital areas when the patient is awake, relaxed, and has his eyes closed. Alpha activity extending over the entire cortex is pathologic in most circumstances. Normal alpha activity should disappear when the patient opens his eyes or attempts complex intellectual tasks, such as multiplication or division [9]. More anteriorly, the electroencepha-

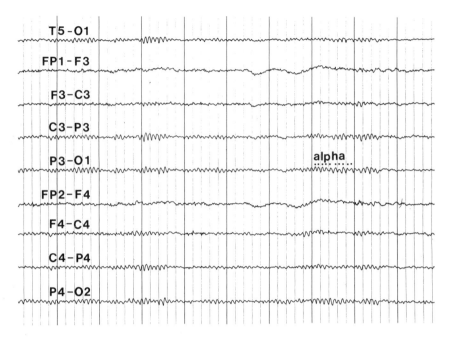

Figure 6–1.
This is a normal adult electroencephalogram obtained while the patient was awake and relaxed with her eyes closed. The most obvious rhythmic activity is alpha activity. The individual waves are marked with dots during the 1-second interval labeled alpha. This patient has alpha-wave activity at a frequency of just under 11 Hz (cycles per second). Alpha activity is clearest in the electrode pairs that include the occipital (O1, O2) or adjacent parietal (P3, P4) regions. (T = temporal; O = occipital; FP = frontoparietal; F = frontal; C = central; P = parietal.)

logram will show irregular combinations of waves at varying frequencies, but very slow waves in the range below 4 Hz should not appear in an adult while he is awake. With drowsiness, the obvious waveforms on the record slow.

The normal electroencephalographic pattern changes with the age of the patient, and patterns that are clearly pathologic at one age may be just normal variants at another age [10]. High-amplitude symmetrical slow waves in the awake infant are normal at some stages of development, even though they suggest structural damage or hydrocephalus in middle-aged adults. Alpha activity slows with age, and so an alpha wave rhythm that slips to 7 Hz at times in an elderly person should arouse no concern. Even focal slowing is common and usually benign in the elderly. Focal slowing of the brain waves to 5 to 6 Hz over one temporal lobe would be worrisome in a 30-year-old person, but it usually is associated with no significant pathology when it appears in a 70-year-old individual [9].

Spikes and slow waves generally are evident when a patient is having a

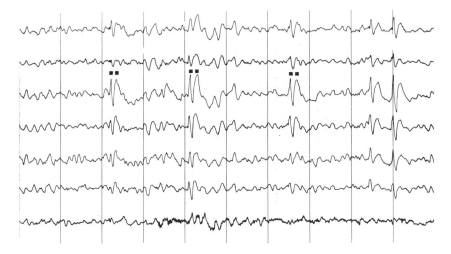

Figure 6–2.
This record from a young boy with intractable seizures shows recurrent spike–and–slow wave discharges (■ ■).

seizure, and individuals with epilepsy routinely have spike or slow wave activity between seizure episodes as well [8, 11]. These are called *epileptiform activity.* Sharp waves and spikes not associated with epilepsy and occurring in an awake individual usually indicate brain damage, but this is not always the case. Epileptiform activity is seen in 2.2 percent of the electroencephalograms recorded from nonepileptic people in the general population [12].

Sharp waves arising from the occipital area are a normal variant in some elderly individuals. Another normal variant is a cluster of spikes that appear to be pointing downward and that occur at a frequency of 14 or 6 cycles per second. These are called *14-* and *6-per-second positive spikes,* and they usually arise in the temporal regions in healthy young adults or adolescents, often during sleep. With arousal from sleep, some normal children have high-voltage wave activity with small notches that resemble spike–and–slow wave activity [13]. The importance of these normal variants is that they can lead to considerable misinterpretation of the electroencephalogram, especially when a seizure is suspected.

Although the electroencephalogram cannot establish the cause of epilepsy, some patterns do limit the possible causes of the brain damage. Periodic spike or sharp wave discharges occurring more than once every 4 seconds may develop with subacute sclerosing panencephalitis, a lethal degenerative disease of the brain. When spikes, sharp waves, or high-voltage slow waves occur regularly once or twice per second, the underlying brain disease may be Creutzfeldt-Jakob disease (a slow viral encephalitis), herpes encephalitis (a more conventional virus affecting people of all ages), or Tay-Sachs disease (an inborn error of metabolism causing dementia in children). With brain damage from poisons or anoxia, a periodic pattern may develop in which wave activity is largely absent between discharges. Such a pattern is called *periodic lateralized epileptiform discharges* (PLED), and it may develop with focal lesions that cause epilepsy [13]. Tumors, strokes, or less obvious structural lesions may produce PLED, and focal seizures often are seen in association with PLED.

Provocative Techniques

Various maneuvers will make abnormal electroencephalographic activity more apparent. Such maneuvers involve manipulating the patient to some extent, but the measures used never pose any danger to the average patient. Obviously, each patient's medical problems must be taken into account before any provocative stimuli are employed. An individual with congestive heart disease should not be expected to hyperventilate, and an individual allergic to a variety of sedatives should not be given those sedatives. The provocative measures are intended to make abnormal brain wave activity more obvious *without* precipitating a seizure.

Sleep

Sleep lowers the seizure threshold, but when the patient goes without sleep for an unusually long interval, the seizure threshold is lowered even more. The physician does not want to precipitate seizures, but by having the patient sleep little the night before testing, or by inducing sleep during the electroencephalographic recording, the physician enhances the likelihood that subtle abnormalities will appear on the electroencephalogram that would not otherwise be evident [13]. This is not frank seizure activity, but it indicates that the patient's sleep state allows abnormal cortical activity to break through.

If the patient cannot relax enough to sleep during the recording, chloral hydrate, 500 to 1,500 mg orally, depending on the size of the patient, may suffice to induce sleep. This drug alters the electroencephalographic record much less than many other sedatives and can be given to children in syrup form. The dose for children should be based on their age and weight or body surface area. Sleep recording is time-consuming, inconvenient and, for most patients, not necessary, but when suspicion of a seizure disorder is high and the patient's electroencephalogram is normal in the awake state, a sleep study should be done.

Hyperventilation

If the patient breathes rapidly and deeply for several minutes, the brain wave patterns will change. Higher-amplitude and lower-frequency waves will appear in normal individuals. In patients with low seizure thresholds, this hyperventilation may unmask the focus of the spike or slow wave activity. Asymmetry, spikes, or sharp waves developing with hyperventilation may help in localizing the cortical problem. Children with generalized absence seizures can predictably induce transient spike-and-wave discharges on the electroencephalogram when they hyperventilate.

Photic Stimulation
Flashing lights trigger seizures in some individuals, but in most, photic stimulation simply elicits electroencephalographic responses that may reveal a subtle focal abnormality [13]. Patients with epilepsy who have seizures on exposure to flashing lights at a certain frequency should not be exposed to these stimuli. If no specific abnormality has been uncovered by a routine electroencephalographic study, photic stimulation may reveal focal spike activity [14].

Special Electrode Placements

To detect spike activity arising on the mesial or inner aspect of the temporal lobe, special electrode arrangements may be required. One electrode intended for this type of recording is the nasopharyngeal lead. This is inserted into the nose and set against the lateral aspect of the nasopharynx so that it lies close to the mesial aspect of the temporal lobe. It is not glued or forced into the mucosa of the nasopharynx, and so it is fairly atraumatic. Most patients can sleep with nasopharyngeal leads in place, allowing the special advantages of a sleep recording to be combined with the advantages of nasopharyngeal leads.

More direct, but more traumatic, approaches to the temporal lobe use sphenoidal or nasoethmoidal electrodes [15]. These alternative electrode placements are most valuable when the routine electrode arrangements yield a normal or ambiguous record in a patient who has signs or symptoms of complex partial epilepsy [13].

Video Monitoring with Electroencephalography

Several techniques have been developed for long-term study of patients with seizures. These include videotaping patients while they are undergoing electroencephalography. Using split-screen video techniques to display the electroencephalogram alongside the simultaneous video record of the patient's behavior, subtle correlations can be made between behavioral and electroencephalographic changes. This approach has been especially helpful in the evaluation of factitious seizures, but it also has found widespread application in the investigation of a variety of infantile and adult seizure disorders [16]. Records of electroencephalographic activity over the course of 24 hours often point to unsuspected patterns of seizure activity or document the absence of electrical abnormalities during repeated factitious seizures. The development of portable recording equipment and telemetric devices has allowed recordings to be obtained from patients while they are active.

Combined video and electroencephalographic monitoring may reveal that the patient with poorly controlled or intractable seizures has a type of epilepsy that was not suspected [16]. Medication changes made on the basis of information provided by these techniques often improve the level of seizure control [16].

Evoked Potential Studies

Combining electroencephalographic techniques and computerized analysis of electrical changes is the basis for evoked cortical potential studies. A repeated stimulus is given to the patient, and short-term brain wave changes induced by the stimulus are monitored. These changes usually are so slight that they become apparent only after many individual evoked potentials are averaged by computer. The recurrent stimulus may be a click for auditory evoked potentials, a shifting checkerboard pattern for visual evoked potentials, or an electrical shock to a peripheral nerve for somatosensory evoked potentials [17]. Each time the stimulus occurs, the electroencephalogram is recorded by a computer. The computer then averages the responses from dozens of stimuli and produces a record of the voltage changes associated with the recurrent stimulus [18].

Evoked cortical potential studies have been used to document changes in sensory pathways to the brain and have found many applications in clinical neurology, but they remain primarily research tools, having few advantages in clinical practice over a thorough neurologic examination. The most obvious advantage of such studies is that they are a means of objectively assessing several different types of primarily subjective phenomena, such as sensation and perception [17]. The results are reproducible, and subtle changes can be detected on repeated examinations. Changes in sensory, motor, and perceptual abilities that might go unnoticed by the patient can be detected with this technique.

COMPUTED TOMOGRAPHY

Computed tomographic scanning of the head uses computer analysis of x-ray absorption to construct an image of the brain in two dimensions (Fig. 6–3). This technique has had an enormous impact on all of neurology [7, 19, 20]. Although it is expensive, it has been widely used in the evaluation of epilepsy. Any individual with seizures of recent onset should be examined with this technique, unless the patient is a pregnant woman with no focal neurologic signs.

Precautions must be observed so that there are no untoward reactions to

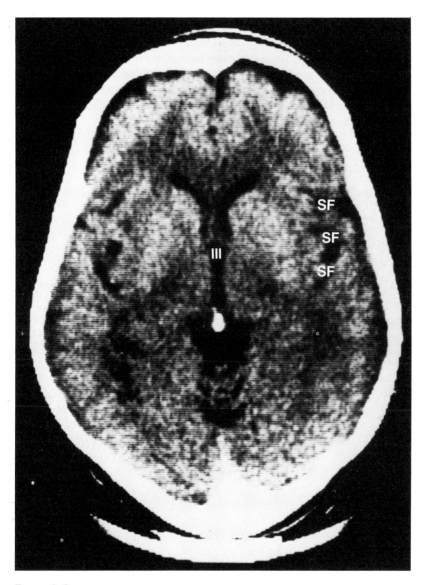

Figure 6–3.
The sylvian fissures (SF) and third ventricle (III) are well visualized on this normal computed tomogram of the head.

the radiographic dye, administered during the study to allow better visualization of the blood vessels in the brain. Patients with renal disease or congestive heart failure may develop fluid overload with infusion of the dye. People with sickle cell disease may also develop complications from the dye if it induces sickling. With complicated migraine, the irritation associated with the dye may induce protracted vasospasm in the head that leads to strokes. Despite these possible complications, computed tomography of the head has proved to be a remarkably benign technique.

OTHER DIAGNOSTIC TOOLS

The selection of other techniques to be used in investigating the patient with apparent seizures is made on an individual basis. Not all patients with seizures should have angiography, but many patients without obvious signs of central nervous system infection should have lumbar punctures to check the cerebrospinal fluid. The patient's history, clinical examination, and initial investigations will determine which additional studies should be carried out.

Routine and Digital Subtraction Angiography

Routine cerebral angiography involves the insertion of a catheter into a major artery, usually the femoral artery, and injection of contrast material once the catheter is in or near the origin of a major intracranial vessel (Fig. 6–4) [7]. There are several limitations and possible complications of this technique. Placing the catheter requires considerable skill and cannot be done rapidly even by experienced hands. Atheromatous material may embolize from the vessel wall as the catheter is manipulated. Even introducing the catheter into the arterial system involves some risk of hemorrhaging in susceptible individuals.

Despite these problems, arteriography has been extremely useful in the investigation of intracranial lesions associated with epilepsy. It is still invaluable in the recognition of small arteriovenous malformations and aneurysms. The investigation of subarachnoid hemorrhage, a potential cause of seizures, invariably requires routine cerebral angiography.

Radiographic materials are much more easily introduced into the venous system, but, until recently, the low concentration of dye that reached the cerebral vessels made such injections useless in evaluating even the largest intracranial vessels. This all changed with the development of digital subtraction angiography, which allows a strictly venous injection of dye to be used for studies of intracranial and extracranial blood vessels (Fig. 6–5). The technique involves fluoroscopy of the cerebral vessels opacified by intravenous contrast media, with image intensification and computerized subtraction of nonvascular structures [21]. Although the resolution of intracranial vessels still is not ad-

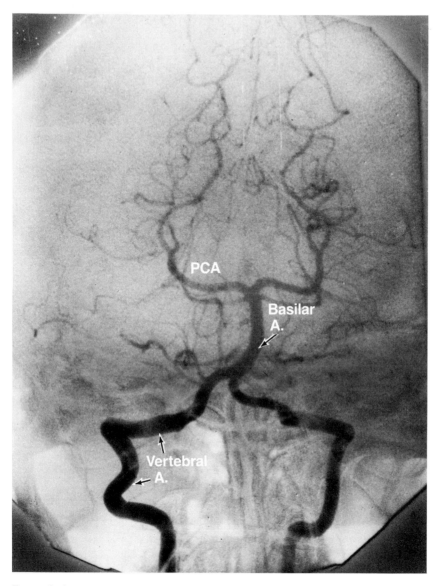

Figure 6–4.
The vertebral arteries (Vertebral A.) and their branches are well visualized on this transfemoral angiogram. The right vertebral artery was selectively catheterized, and the left was filled with dye by retrograde flow of the contrast material. The basilar artery (Basilar A.) and posterior cerebral artery (PCA) are normal. The skull has been subtracted from the image by strictly photographic techniques.

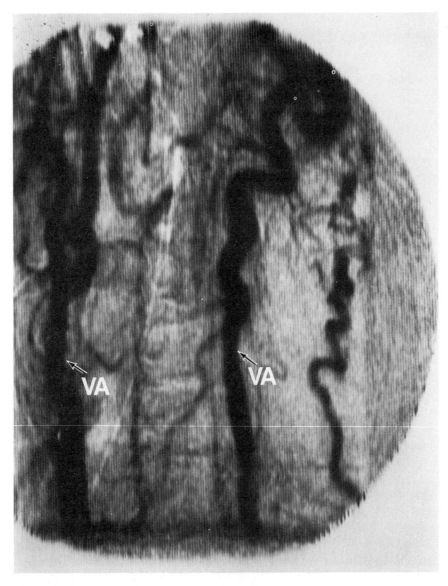

Figure 6–5.
The vertebral arteries (VA) are well defined on this digital subtraction angiogram of the neck, because there are few other vessels filled with contrast media. This patient had complete occlusion of the left carotid artery and partial occlusion of the right carotid artery.

equate for many presurgical studies and the level of patient cooperation for a useful study must be high, digital subtraction angiography provides good resolution of vascular abnormalities in the head and neck.

Digital subtraction angiography eliminates the risk of hemorrhage from arterial puncture, can be performed on outpatients, and generally costs half as much as a conventional arteriography [21]. Aside from allergic reactions to the dye, the main complications of this technique are acute pulmonary edema and renal failure, both of which are rare and may be avoided by limiting the amount of contrast medium used in individuals with poor cardiac or renal function [21].

Lumbar Puncture

Lumbar puncture to obtain spinal fluid for examination is one of the oldest and most useful neurologic tools available to the physician [2]. This procedure must be performed whenever there is reason to suspect a central nervous system infection, and it is helpful in investigating other problems that may cause seizures [22]. The patient with a normal computed tomogram and abruptly appearing seizures may have a subarachnoid hemorrhage, meningeal carcinomatosis, or meningeal lymphomatosis, all of which usually require spinal fluid studies for their identification.

With a lumbar puncture, the physician has an opportunity to measure directly the intracranial pressure, as well as to check the cerebrospinal fluid for elevated protein or depressed glucose contents. With a cerebral vasculitis, such as that occurring in lupus cerebritis, the only apparent abnormalities on neurologic evaluation may be an unusual brain wave pattern on the electroencephalogram and elevated protein content in the cerebrospinal fluid [4]. Cerebrospinal fluid cultures may be supplemented by studies of cryptococcal antigen to assess the possibility of cryptococcal infection, staining of the fluid to look for bacteria and fungi, and cytologic evaluation of the fluid to look for cancer or lymphoma cells. Immunoglobulin electrophoresis has been of practical value primarily in the study of demyelinating diseases, nervous system disorders that do not usually cause seizures.

Magnetic Resonance Imaging

Magnetic resonance imaging provides a view of brain anatomy that promises to be even more revealing than computed tomography, and it uses magnetic fields, rather than ionizing radiation, to determine brain structure. A computer analyzes information provided by the application of a magnetic field to determine several structural and physiologic properties of the organ being studied. This technique, in its simplest form, analyzes water content of the tissue in the magnetic field. Bony structures are largely invisible on magnetic resonance studies, and so conventional subtraction techniques are unnecessary. The equipment is still very expensive and the long-term effects of exposure to the magnetic fields remains to be established. However, experience with magnetic fields in other settings suggests that there will be no problems with widespread application of this technique.

Positron Emission Tomography

Positron emission tomography uses radioactive materials to reveal metabolic changes in the brain in very limited areas. An array of radiation detectors is placed around the head and, with computer assistance, emissions from positron-emitting radionuclides can be localized. Fluorine 18, nitrogen 13, oxygen 15, and carbon 11 are the most commonly used substances, with ^{18}F-labeled 2-fluorodeoxyglucose currently finding the most applications [23]. It has been used to study patients with epilepsy, and the findings have been provocative and reproducible. During the interictal period, the positron emission tomogram may reveal an area of hypometabolism corresponding to the epileptogenic focus. During a seizure, this same area may have an increased level of metabolic activity [23]. Practical applications of this technique include the localization of seizure foci prior to surgery and the documentation of epileptic activity in patients with ambiguous electroencephalograms [23]. Positron emission tomography still is strictly experimental and will probably see much less practical application than nuclear magnetic resonance.

Brain Biopsy

In some patients, the epilepsy remains unexplained after all reasonable studies of the nervous system have been attempted. If the patient's condition is deteriorating and a life-threatening disorder is suspected, a brain biopsy may help in diagnosis and treatment. However, this is a neurosurgical procedure that necessarily injures the cerebral cortex and so provides a focus for seizure activity if the patient recovers from his underlying disease. Brain biopsy is a more routine investigation when a mass is evident on other studies. The biopsy will allow histologic identification of the mass so that any tumor, granuloma, abscess, or hamartoma that is found may be managed while antiepileptic medication is given. If the biopsy reveals intracellular inclusions that suggest a hereditary metabolic disease, the patient may not be helped but the family will be spared a great deal of uncertainty and the need for further manipulation of the patient.

INVESTIGATIVE RESTRAINT

Determining which tests should not be performed in the investigation of the patient with epilepsy is often a major concern of the physician responsible for the patient. In some settings, such as that in which the patient is a neonate who had several seizures during its first 2 days of life, the course of investigation is generally agreed on and largely obligatory. In the older child or adult who has only one or a few seizures, it is much more controversial and the physician usually faces less urgency. Many neurologists would not perform a lumbar puncture on a 12-year-old who has just had a generalized convulsion, but most neurologists would want a thorough examination of the cerebrospinal fluid of a 20-year-old patient who has just had his first seizure. The probability that the epilepsy is idiopathic obviously plays a large role in deciding how limited the investigation of the patient will be, but what may appear to be idiopathic epilepsy may prove to be seizures associated with chronic meningitis.

In general, the physician must be guided by his or her overall impression of the patient's current condition and the risk of complications. If the adolescent has generalized seizures and no neurologic deficits interictally, there is no justification for obtaining an angiogram and little reason to do a lumbar puncture. Electroencephalography is appropriate and computed tomography is justifiable, but the probability that this is an idiopathic generalized seizure is so great if the child is passing through puberty that more attention to treatment and less to investigations is reasonable. The 40-year-old man who has his first seizure must be considered at high risk for meningitis or tumor, and so more invasive studies, such as lumbar puncture and angiography, will be performed without hesitation on this patient.

In every case, the physician must be influenced by the initial neurologic examination, the patient's past history, and the feasibility of observing the patient for weeks or months. In a rural community, it may be practical to limit the investigation of a patient who appears asymptomatic after a seizure that occurred with alcohol abuse or a viral syndrome. In the more chaotic setting of the urban clinic, such a patient may require hospitalization to allow investigation of symptoms that might otherwise prove devastating if they progressed while the patient was unavailable for further study and treatment. Those investigative methods that should be a routine part of a patient's evaluation must be selected on the basis of the primary physician's own experience with the types of patients that present themselves.

REFERENCES

1. Denny-Brown, D. *Handbook of Neurological Examination and Case Recording.* Cambridge, Mass.: Harvard University Press, 1967.
2. DeJong, R.N. *The Neurologic Examination.* New York: Harper & Row, 1979.
3. Lechtenberg, R. *The Psychiatrist's Guide to Diseases of the Nervous System.* New York: John Wiley & Sons, 1982.
4. Merritt, H.H. *A Textbook of Neurology,* ed. 6. Philadelphia: Lea & Febiger, 1979.
5. Hartmann, E. Sleep. In Nicholi, A.M. (ed.), *The Harvard Guide to Modern Psychiatry.* Cambridge, Mass.: Belknap Press, 1978, p. 103.

6. Volpe, J.J. Neonatal seizures. *Clin. Perinatol.* 4(1):43–63, 1977.
7. Adams, R.D., Victor, M. *Principles of Neurology,* ed. 2. New York: McGraw-Hill, 1981.
8. Gastaut, H. Clinical and electroencephalographical classification of epileptic seizures. *Epilepsia* 11:102, 1970.
9. Harner, R.N. EEG evaluation of the patient with dementia. In Benson, D.F., Blumer, D. (eds.), *Psychiatric Aspects of Neurologic Disease.* New York: Grune & Stratton, 1975, p. 63.
10. Kaszniak, A.W., Garron, D.C., Fox, J.H., et al. Cerebral atrophy, EEG slowing, age, education, and cognitive functioning in suspected dementia. *Neurology* (N.Y.) 29:1273, 1979.
11. Goldensohn, E.S. The classification of epileptic seizures. In Tower, D.B. (ed.), *The Nervous System,* vol. 2. New York: Raven Press, 1975, p. 261.
12. Zivin, L., Ajmone-Marsan, C. Incidence and prognostic significance of "epileptiform" activity in the EEG of non-epileptic subjects. *Brain* 91:751–758, 1968.
13. Goldensohn, E., Koehle, R. *EEG Interpretation.* Mt. Kisco, N.Y.: Futura Publishing Co., 1975, p. 186.
14. Hauser, W.A., Anderson, V.E., Loewenson, R.B., et al. Seizure recurrence after a first unprovoked seizure. *N. Engl. J. Med.* 307(9):522–528, 1982.
15. Schomer, D.L. Partial epilepsy. *N. Engl. J. Med.* 309(9):536–539, 1983.
16. Theodore, W.H., Schulman, E.A., Porter, R.J. Intractable seizures: long-term follow-up after prolonged inpatient treatment in an epilepsy unit. *Epilepsia* 24(3):336–343, 1983.
17. Chiappa, K.H., Ropper, A.H. Evoked potentials in clinical medicine (part 2). *N. Engl. J. Med.* 306(20):1205–1211, 1982.
18. Anziska, B., Cracco, R.Q. Short latency somatosensory evoked potentials: studies in patients with focal neurological disease. *Electroencephalogr. Clin. Neurophysiol.* 49:227, 1980.
19. Jacobson, R.L., Farmer, T.W. The "hypernormal" CT scan in dementia: bilateral isodense subdural hematomas. *Neurology* (N.Y.) 29:1522, 1979.
20. Owens, D.G., Johnstone, E.C., Bydder, M., et al. Unsuspected organic disease in chronic schizophrenia demonstrated by computed tomography. *J. Neurol. Neurosurg. Psychiatry* 43:1065, 1980.
21. Intravenous digital subtraction angiography. *Med. Lett. Drugs Ther.* 25(649):107–108, 1983.
22. Korein, J., Cravioto, H., Leicach, M. Reevaluation of lumbar puncture. *Neurology* (N.Y.) 9:290, 1959.
23. Engel, J., Jr., Troupin, A.S., Crandall, P.H., et al. Recent developments in the diagnosis and therapy of epilepsy. *Ann. Intern. Med.* 97:584–598, 1982.

7. Adults with Epilepsy

Physical and psychological traits of the patient with epilepsy, the type of epilepsy he or she has, and the extent to which the seizures can be controlled with medication all influence the impact of epilepsy on the affected adult. With effective treatment, many adults with epilepsy are virtually unrestricted in their daily routines and long-term goals. If seizures occur infrequently or do not occur at all, work, recreation, sexual activity, family interactions, and athletic activities will be fairly normal for the person with epilepsy. Unfortunately, many adults with epilepsy are burdened with frequent seizures or the threat of seizures. Familiarity with the neurologic problem does not reduce its impact, regardless of the age of the patient when seizures first appear. The family practitioner, internist, gynecologist, or neurologist primarily responsible for the patient's welfare can minimize the disruptiveness of the epilepsy by anticipating problems that will be encountered and by developing strategies to help the patient avoid these problems.

SOCIAL ADJUSTMENT

Adjusting to epilepsy means working, relaxing, and striving for goals with as much confidence and as much success as the average person without epilepsy. Most individuals with epilepsy do adjust fairly well in both practical and social terms. Factors contributing to poor social adjustment include poor seizure control, intellectual impairment, personality disorders, generalized convulsive seizures, seizures secondary to head trauma, brain tumors, or encephalitis, and easily provoked seizures. Relatively normal life-styles are exhibited by 92 percent of patients with seizures not associated with any intellectual or personality disorders [1]. These people are not free of problems, but the social difficulties they face are surmountable. There are several factors that predictably enter into an individual's adjustment to epilepsy. How well a patient copes is closely related to how well controlled the seizures are and how unimpaired that person is by other neurologic problems [1]. The effort required to overcome social and practical problems, such as isolation from friends, discrimination on the job, and exclusion from some sports, obviously varies considerably with the type of seizure disorder, the level of control achieved, and the social milieu of the patient.

Each person with epilepsy usually has a few special concerns that overshadow other problems incited by the seizure disorder. Many adults with epilepsy worry about the impact the disorder has on other family members. The distress that they cause their families is a common concern of patients with poorly controlled seizures. They see their families as victims of this disorder [2], as much as they see themselves as victims of the epilepsy. More than half admit that they have considerable difficulty accepting that they have a neurologic disorder [3].

The patients who most often exhibit poor social adjustment are those with dementia or psychological disturbances as well as seizures. Even with a personality disorder, as many as 52 percent of people with epilepsy have a normal social adjustment [1]. Intellectual impairment more seriously limits the patient's adjustment to epilepsy. Only 21 percent of people with dementia or mental retardation and epilepsy have a fairly normal social adjustment. With both intellectual and personality disorders in the same patient, this is reduced to 15 percent [1].

The type of epilepsy the patient has determines in part whether a relatively normal life-style can be achieved. Epilepsies in which the seizures have few clinical signs are those that are the least disruptive socially. A normal adjustment occurs in 87 percent of patients with generalized absence seizures, regardless of their other problems [1]. Individuals with generalized tonic-clonic seizures caused by head trauma, brain tumors, or encephalitis often exhibit poor social adjustments [1].

The frequency of seizures also influences the extent to which a normal life-style can be achieved [4]. For most patients, the likelihood of normal social adjustment is slightly better than the likelihood of complete seizure control for each type of epilepsy. Eighty-four percent of patients whose seizures are fully controlled with medication make normal adjustments [1]. In contrast, only 38 percent achieve social normalcy if seizures are not fully controlled and medication changes fail to improve the level of control [1]. Even patients with intellectual or emotional problems will be better socially adjusted with improved seizure control [4].

Despite the advantages of improved seizure control, in some cases it is the antiepileptic regimen itself that interferes with adjustment and productivity. If the patient is toxic from the medication, that person will not be able to function optimally even if seizure control is excellent [4]. A balance must be reached between the most beneficial dose of drugs for seizure control and the highest dose that can be tolerated by the patient.

No one can confidently predict the level of function that a person with epilepsy is capable of achieving, but the physician familiar with the epileptic adult's limitations is ultimately responsible for setting the goals to be reached. What is feasible will be determined, in large part, by the affected individual's intellectual abilities and personality traits, as well as his level of seizure control. An accurate appraisal of the patient's talents and limitations will contribute to his realizing that potential and will help minimize the frustration likely to develop from pressure to achieve unreasonable goals.

Provocative Stimuli

Sleep deprivation, physical exhaustion, trauma, infection, and alcohol abuse are common causes of recurrent seizures in individuals with well-controlled epilepsy, but the commonest cause is erratic antiepileptic drug use. All of these provocative situations and stimuli must be avoided if the risk of seizures is to be minimized. For most people, this means developing daily routines to avoid irregular hours, excessive fatigue, and lapses in personal hygiene.

Less common, but more disturbing, are seizures triggered by common and largely unavoidable stimuli in the environment. If the seizures are almost always initiated by a particular stimulus and do not appear unless that stimulus is present, the seizure pattern may be called *reflex epilepsy*. The stimulus that triggers a seizure need be nothing more than a specific smell, noise, sight, or action [5]. Even eating or looking to one side may initiate seizures [5]. With experience, most patients will learn what triggers their seizures and will avoid those provocative stimuli.

The common concern that emotional distress will provoke seizures is exaggerated. Emotional stress rarely triggers seizures, even in people with low seizure thresholds [6]. Identifying those stimuli that cause increased seizure activity is valuable in improving seizure control when other measures to suppress seizure activity are being pursued, but trying to eliminate emotional stress from the environment of the adult with epilepsy may be more disturbing than the stress itself. Minimizing the emotional demands on a patient isolates that patient.

Guilt

People with epilepsy often feel personally responsible for the neurologic disorder. This guilt is especially obvious in accident victims, even when they suffered injuries as innocent bystanders. The combination of this guilt and feelings of worthlessness that often develop when epilepsy limits the individual's acitivities can lead to depression and self-destructive behavior. Aggravating the guilt is the embarrassment that some patients feel when the seizures occur in public. This is beyond logical explanation, since these same people will feel no guilt or embarrassment on suffering a myocardial infarction or breaking a leg in public. Family and friends often reinforce the patient's sense of responsibility by insisting that he or she brings on seizures by not taking suitable preventive measures. This inappropriate sense of responsibility often interferes with social adjustment.

Isolation

As the epilepsy becomes a chronic health problem, many victims of the disorder withdraw from family, friends, and colleagues [7]. Even the relationships that survive the patient's withdrawal often become strained or awkward. Friendships, family ties, and patient-doctor relationships that persist in the face of chronic neurologic problems often are sheltered by the individual with epilepsy from anger, abuse, or even assertiveness [7]. The relationships become too valuable to threaten with normal conflicts. Dependence on a spouse may be total. The epileptic individual's isolation and dependence may breed antagonism toward those on whom he is dependent, and this anger fosters more isolation from long-standing friends and colleagues.

Employment

Twenty-one percent of adults with epilepsy believe that the greatest problem they face is finding and maintaining employment [8]. Although the outlook is not as grim as many people believe, there certainly are employment problems. Individuals having the most difficulty securing and staying in jobs are those with both epilepsy and intellectual impairment [9]. The severity of epileptic attacks correlates, to some extent, with employment, a finding which suggests that real disability, rather than prejudice, is important in determining overall employment rates for adults with epilepsy [10, 11]. However, the type of epilepsy and the frequency of attacks generally do not correlate with the probability of being employed [12]. When unemployment levels approach 3 or 4 percent, the adult with seizures that are well controlled, who has a good education and no health problems other than epilepsy, can expect to have nearly the same chance of securing a job as the individual without seizures [10]. Patients with frequent disabling attacks have an unemployment rate of approximately 50 percent [12]. The epileptic person who is most likely to have steady employment is the one who is married, has few or no emotional problems, has been educated beyond high school, and has performed well in school [12].

More than 40 percent of people with epilepsy who have problems securing a job believe that they are turned away on the basis of their neurologic disorder alone [8]. Consequently, approximatley 62 percent of people with epilepsy applying for work will deny having the seizure disorder [8]. This obviously leaves them vulnerable to dismissal if the epilepsy is discovered after they have been hired. When unemployment is high for the general population, people with epilepsy are preferentially excluded from the work force [10]. Approximately 30 percent of patients who lose their jobs are fired shortly after a seizure occurs at work [8].

Employers justify this discrimination by insisting that people with epilepsy are accident-prone and that most work is too hazardous for them. Some employers believe that to hire people with epilepsy they would need facilities to treat the individual who has seizures on the job, and that seizures occurring on the job not only would reduce the productivity of the person with epilepsy, but also would disrupt the work of fellow employees [8, 10]. These fears are not substantiated by work statistics [10].

Absenteeism, injuries, and productivity are about the same for adults with epilepsy as for those without epilepsy. In manufacturing, where the risks associated with epilepsy are presumed to be greatest, performance by individuals with epilepsy is slightly better than that by individuals with no chronic health problems [8]. The better than average safety performance of people with epilepsy reflects a high level of self-regulation. Thirty-seven percent of adults with epilepsy claim that their choice of work was influenced by the fact that they had seizures [8].

Patients who have regular employment and do not conceal their epilepsy lose their jobs usually because of poor performance rather than any problem with the epilepsy. The most important factor influencing whether a person with epilepsy holds onto a job is the patient's psychological function. Patients with long-standing emotional problems, including drug addicts and other patients with personality disorders, usually do not maintain steady employment [12].

The amount of time an individual has been unemployed during the 2 years prior to starting a new job is somewhat indicative of the likelihood that he will stay with the job. The patient who has been out of work for more than 17 of the prior 24 months is not likely to work for very long, regardless of how accommodating the employer is [12].

Hospitalization

Frequent or protracted hospitalizations may interfere with social adjustment, but such hospitalizations still are fairly common. When seizure control is poor, hospitalization may be required to provide a more structured environment and to make dramatic changes in antiepileptic medications. The hospital confinement also provides an opportunity to investigate the basis for the deterioration in seizure control.

Frequent hospitalizations disrupt work, education, and family life, yet hospitalization rates for all types of epilepsies have increased over recent years [13]. In part, this reflects the aging of the population on antiepileptic drugs. As people with epilepsy get older, they are hospitalized more frequently for problems related to their seizure disorders, such as aspiration and injuries [13]. Women are hospitalized more often than men by a factor of approximately 7 percent, a difference that undoubtedly reflects social factors, since the types of epilepsy and severity of the problems faced by patients of each sex are not significantly different [13, 14]. These social factors probably include the more limited economic consequences of hospitalizing a person not working outside the home.

Hospitalization should be the last resort in management of a seizure disorder. The most important goal in treating any type of epilepsy is to fully control the seizures in a normal environment. The dramatic difference between the hospital environment and the home or work environment often is demonstrated by the cessation of all seizure activity after an individual is simply removed from his usual surroundings. The change in environment is sufficient, without any change in medication, but the benefits of hospitalization often are annulled as soon as the patient is discharged from the hospital.

COPING WITH COINCIDENTAL PROBLEMS

For some people, epilepsy is merely one facet of a nervous system disease that produces several disabilities. Seizures may be associated with mental retardation and clumsiness in individuals with perinatal hypoxia, or with paralysis and speech disorders in individuals who have suffered strokes. In many patients with extensive nervous system damage, the epilepsy is a relatively minor feature of the central nervous system disease.

Paralysis

Weakness in a limb or a hemiparesis occasionally develops after a seizure, a transient phenomenon called *postictal* or *Todd paralysis*, but many patients with structural brain damage have both seizures and focal weakness or spasticity from the central nervous system injury. That central nervous system injury may be a progressive lesion from a tumor or vascular malformation, or it may be a static lesion associated with trauma, a stroke, or perinatal asphyxia. If an apparently static lesion produces new signs, the individual must be reinvestigated for a progressive lesion. Occasionally, a person with hemiparesis and seizures will develop more frequent seizures with no change in the hemiparesis. That the focal neurologic signs have not changed does not necessarily mean that the responsible lesion has remained static, but it does increase the likelihood that the problem is a change in compliance with antiepileptic regimens or an altered pattern of drug metabolism.

Dementia

Some individuals with intellectual impairment also have epilepsy, and approximately 15 percent of patients with seizure disorders are intellectually impaired [8]. Their dementia varies from slight memory problems to profound mental retardation, and in some cases, the intellectual impairment is the individual's principal difficulty. Because mental retardation is generally from structural or metabolic injuries to the cerebral cortex, fully 60 percent of the mentally retarded have some type of seizure disorder [8].

Some individuals without apparent cerebral damage but with epilepsy have cognitive deficits, such as poor memory or language difficulties. Among patients with no other obvious handicaps or illnesses who are socially well-adjusted, there is a subtle but consistent impairment in short-term and long-term memory [15]. The degree of impairment does not correlate with the frequency of the seizures, the type of epilepsy, the number of years the patient has had the epilepsy, or the type of antiepileptic drug the patient takes [15]. The significance of the defect becomes apparent as the individual enters adult life, but it is not more apparent if the patient developed epilepsy in early childhood rather than adolescence. In fact, the patients with the most obvious memory problems are those who developed the epilepsy during adolescence [15].

The apparent focus for seizure activity affects the severity of memory disturbances in patients with epilepsy. A temporal lobe focus producing complex partial seizures causes more impairment than foci elsewhere in the cortex that produce simple partial seizures [15]. The severity of the impairment over the course of years is not affected by the patient's use or avoidance of any antiepileptic drug. Antiepileptics may exacerbate the memory difficulty transiently, but this is more often a sign of toxicity than an effect of therapeutic levels.

Electroencephalographic findings in patients with epilepsy and severe memory impairment suggest that subtle features of the epilepsy determine its influence on intellectual function. Patients with interictal spike-and-wave complexes on the electroencephalogram have the most difficulty on tests of recall [15]. The side of the seizure focus or the interictal activity plays no role in determining the severity of memory impairment.

Vulnerability to Other Diseases

Poorly controlled seizures pose health risks for the individual with epilepsy. Pneumonia may develop if the person with epilepsy aspirates during a seizure, and the person with epilepsy may exhibit an impaired resistance to aspiration pneumonia, which will complicate recovery. This is especially true in individuals with congenital brain damage and degenerative central nervous system diseases. More strictly traumatic injuries are common with generalized tonic-clonic seizures. Violent muscle contractions may collapse vertebrae or dislocate shoulders. When the patient falls or bangs a limb against hard surfaces, fractures in the long bones may occur.

SEXUAL ACTIVITY

Sexual activity is normal in most people with epilepsy. Notable exceptions include those patients with complex partial epilepsy and poor seizure control [16]. In most instances in which sexual function is abnormal, the main problem is a lack of interest. Compounding the problem is the fear that sexual intercourse or just excitement will cause seizures. This concern is more likely to inhibit the sexual partners of people with epilepsy rather than the individuals with epilepsy themselves. Sexual eccentricities, such as transvestitism and fetishism, occur with a slightly higher than expected incidence in the population suffering from complex partial epilepsy, but they still are rare.

Controlling seizures often, but not always, minimizes the sexual problems that seem to evolve along with the epilepsy. Unfortunately, some antiepileptic drugs can cause sexual problems of their own, such as impotence and cosmetic changes. Skin and periodontal problems caused by these drugs may undermine the individual's self-confidence or detract from his or her appearance.

Hyposexuality

The major sexual problem faced by couples who engage in regular sexual activity is the anxiety fostered by the epilepsy when seizure control is poor. Improved seizure control will usually eliminate this problem, but that solution may be elusive. When seizure control is not feasible, alternatives must be found to minimize the impact of recurrent seizures.

The alternative approach that usually is most effective is explaining to the sexual partners that the techniques they use during sexual intercourse pose no special threat even if a seizure occurs. The altered breathing pattern, strained expression, and stiffening of limbs that ordinarily accompany sexual excitement in both men and women are often too reminiscent of seizure phenomena for the sexual partners to fully relax and allow excitement to lead to orgasm. Eliminating this inhibition is difficult with even the most unguarded of couples, but it is impossible with couples who cannot talk frankly or accurately about their sexual problems and techniques. If the physician is uncomfortable managing this type of problem, it is best to involve a sex therapist who can be more candid and relaxed [17].

Individuals with complex partial epilepsy have more than the expected incidence of sexual problems. Decreased sexual activity—that is, hyposexuality—is the commonest problem, although most people with complex partial epilepsy do not complain about their lack of sexual activity. Rather, complaints about hyposexuality usually originate in the affected individual's sexual partner. Impotence and frigidity occur in as many as 50 percent of people with complex partial epilepsy, as compared to 30 percent of individuals with generalized tonic-clonic epilepsy and other chronic medical illnesses [16].

Patients with hyposexuality do not develop new sexual preferences.

Homosexuality and pederasty as manifestations of any type of epilepsy, including epilepsy secondary to temporal lobe damage, have never been convincingly demonstrated [18–22]. Individuals with complex partial seizures and hyposexuality exhibit a lack of interest in sexual activity of any sort.

The hyposexuality appears to have more psychologic than physiologic bases [20, 23, 24]. The men are not physiologically impotent, and the women do not have dyspareunia (pain with intercourse); they simply fail to initiate or pursue any kind of sexual activity, heterosexual or homosexual. If complex partial seizures start before or at puberty, these individuals often remain without sexual experience or partners throughout their lives [16]. If the seizures start later in life, after a sexual relationship has become well established, the patient's sexual partner usually will complain of the deterioration in sexual interest.

Most people do not realize that epilepsy affects sexual interest, and they remain skeptical when that is offered as the explanation for a change. The person with the epilepsy often suspects that the antiepileptic medication causes the change in libido, whereas the patient's sexual partner routinely suspects that the person with epilepsy is still sexually active, but with another mate. These conjectures lead to obvious problems with drug compliance and decreased trust between the partners.

Occasionally, the antiepileptic is responsible for poor sexual performance by men. Phenobarbital and primidone are associated with an increased incidence of impotence. Phenytoin causes impotence less frequently. When the man with epilepsy has no loss of libido or evidence of peripheral neuropathy that might explain his impotence, a change in medication is appropriate. Replacing phenobarbital with valproic acid or primidone with carbamazepine may eliminate the impotence.

There are other sexual problems that develop in people with epilepsy which are unrelated to the seizure disorder or its treatment. If an individual with long-standing epilepsy has impaired sexual function without impaired interest, the seizure disorder probably is not responsible for the dysfunction. All men with impotence and all women with dyspareunia shoud be investigated for possible causes of these sexual dysfunctions, such as local infections, diabetes mellitus, amyloidosis, and alcoholism [17, 25, 26].

Good seizure control can improve an individual's sexual activity even if other problems are responsible in part for the sexual dysfunction. With the risk of untimely seizures minimized, it is easier for the epileptic individual to enjoy sexual encounters. Full seizure control may also improve libido and performance in some of these patients, another indication that the seizures themselves underlie some of the behavioral changes that are observed [16].

In some patients, especially those who develop complex partial seizures prior to puberty, sexual interest never develops. With early-onset of complex partial epilepsy, sexual interest may not appear even after decades of seizure control [16]. This is not a major problem for these patients, because they do not complain of sexual deprivation and do not seek relationships that are sexually demanding. However, conflicts may arise if this sexually indifferent person marries a sexually active individual. All that can be offered to the frustrated spouse is a frank assessment of his or her position. The sexual interest of the individual with complex partial seizures is not likely to improve, and so the spouse must decide whether this sexually barren relationship is adequately gratifying in other areas to justify continuing it.

Sexual Eccentricities

Patients with complex partial seizures also have more than the expected incidence of fetishism, exhibitionism, and transvestitism [21, 22, 24, 27]. If the seizures do not begin until after adolescence, this type of aberrant sexual behavior may be absent until years after the development of conventional sexual interests. What induces these eccentricities is unknown [24]. The aberrant behavior is not caused by seizure activity: The patient has no altered consciousness or memory impairment during the episode of aberrant sexual activity.

There are also rare patients who exhibit atypical sexual behavior during the aura or the ictus of complex partial seizures [21, 28]. These patients usually are female, and their recall of the behavior is poor [21]. Automatisms occurring as part of the aura or even during the ictus of the seizure may include undressing, masturbation, or attempts at sexual stimulation of people nearby [21]. This rare pattern of behavior may be in dramatic contrast to the individual's usual sexual behavior [28]. Men with these sexual phenomena occasionally have protracted erections (priapism), but they do not commit sexual attacks or other purposeful sexual advances [28].

Seizure activity originating in or associated with long-standing damage to one or both temporal lobes seems to be responsible for the pervasive changes in sexual activity of some individuals with complex partial seizures. It has not been determined whether this is a reversible phenomenon or a permanent side effect of complex partial seizures. Deviant, or at least atypical, sexual behavior is observed more often in individuals with temporal lobe lesions that develop before 3 years of age than it is in the general population [22]. Since the social definition of normal sexual behavior is constantly under revision, all that can be deduced from this observation is that individuals with early temporal lobe damage express different sexual preferences in comparison with their peers [17]. This difference may be reflected simply as less inhibited answers to sexual questionnaires rather than truly different behavior.

Seizures with Sexual Activity

Some women with complex partial seizures experience sexual arousal or orgasm as part of their seizures [21]. This is exceedingly rare even in women and probably never occurs in men. The few men that notice changes in genital sensation about the time of a seizure routinely complain of unerotic or unpleasant sensations [21]. In the few women affected, these orgasmic seizures usually occur premenstrually.

During the postictal and early interictal periods, the affected woman feels sexually satisfied. When the orgasm occurs during the aura of the seizure, the patient can recall it vividly [21]. Sometimes pleasurable sensations in the groin area and vaginal discharge characteristic of sexual excitation occur during the aura, but no orgasm follows.

Some women with this type of seizure disorder allow their antiepileptic drug compliance to lapse so that these orgasmic seizures can break through [21]. These sexual seizures do not occur in prepubertal girls, and in most cases, the woman who exhibits them has a seizure focus in the right temporal lobe [21]. That the sexual feelings are temporal lobe phenomena is supported by reports from neurosurgeons who find that stimulation deep in the temporal lobe of women during operations to manage poorly controlled seizures elicits similar responses [21].

Cosmetic Effects of Antiepileptics

Contributing to the social and sexual problems of young people with epilepsy are the cosmetic effects of antiepileptic treatment. This has been a problem since bromides were introduced for the management of seizures. Triple bromide salts, which are still used occasionally by pediatric neurologists when other antiepileptic agents fail, cause severe acne. The drugs that have replaced this antiepileptic may also cause disturbing skin changes.

Patients sensitive to any antiepileptic medication may develop rashes that range from erythematous to exfoliative. In most cases, this allergic reaction is adequate grounds for discontinuing the medication, but some patients who have fairly mild skin reactions to highly effective antiepileptics are continued on the drugs, an undesirable but occasionally unavoidable approach. Nonallergic reactions may be no less disturbing. Phenytoin and, to a lesser extent, phenobarbital will coarsen facial skin and darken facial hair. Arm and leg hair will also darken and thicken, but this is much less a cosmetic problem than facial hair for young women with epilepsy. The use of valproic acid may cause weight gain or hair loss in some patients. Both men and women develop gingival hyperplasia with phenytoin and phenobarbital use, but which patients will develop noticeable gingival changes with associated tooth loss is unpredictable (Fig. 7–1).

These cosmetic problems cannot be ignored, because without control of these side effects, drug compliance suffers. Many patients would rather risk occasional seizures than have gingival hyperplasia and tooth loss. A change of medication may avoid further skin, hair, and gum problems, but the existing cosmetic changes will not disappear without some type of intervention. The gingival hyperplasia will resolve with extensive gingivectomies and rigorous

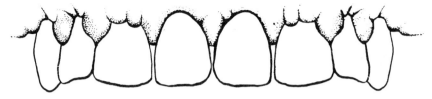

Figure 7–1.
With gingival hyperplasia, the gingiva extends over the teeth and produces a space between the teeth and gums in which debris can accumulate. Periodontal disease will develop unless repeated gingivectomies are performed.

dental care. The limb hair may require shaving or chemical removal if its appearance disturbs the patient. Electrolysis, which permanently removes hair and leaves no stubble, usually is required for removal of facial hair.

PROGNOSIS

Patients with epilepsy have good reason to worry about the long-term prognosis of their neurologic disorder. Insurance companies tell them, through exclusion from policies and exorbitant rates, that epilepsy places them at increased risk of early death. Equally inaccurate notions provided by friends include reports of miraculous cures after a few months of special diets, chiropractic, acupuncture, or other fads. The prognosis is actually different with different types of epilepsy and is affected by systemic or other neurologic problems associated with the seizure disorder.

Remission

That a remission has occurred with epilepsy is difficult to establish, since epilepsy may be inactive for several years before recurring. True remission means that the person no longer has an abnormally low seizure threshold and does not need antiepileptic medication to suppress seizure activity. In fact, most seizures that develop or persist after adolescence do not remit. This is especially true if the patient's electroencephalograms reveal abnormalities in one or both anterior temporal lobes [9]. The prognostic significance of this pattern is important simply because there is no consensus that other patterns observed in adults correlate with the likelihood of continued seizure activity or remission. The complex partial seizures associated with these anterior temporal lobe abnormalities will require medication for decades and often will still be poorly controlled [9].

Even when antiepileptic medication has been effective in suppressing seizure activity for decades, the patient usually will have recurrent seizures if the med-

Table 7–1.
Risk of Seizure Recurrence when Drugs Are Stopped after Protracted Seizure
Control

Seizure Type	Recurrence Rate (%)
Generalized nonconvulsive	5–25
Simple partial	25
Generalized tonic-clonic	60–80
Nonconvulsive and tonic-clonic	65
Juvenile myoclonic	75–95

ication is stopped (Table 7–1) [29]. This is very different from the natural history of epilepsy in children, in whom seizures often remit as they mature, even if the electroencephalogram remains abnormal after the seizures have been well controlled for years (see Chapter 10) [9, 29].

Rehabilitation

After an adult develops seizures, rehabilitation is often appropriate. If the seizure disorder develops after the individual has been involved in a stable family and job, both may be severely disrupted. Rehabilitation is most appropriate in managing problems with employment, interpersonal relationships, and self-esteem. This may mean training the patient for a new job or involving the individual in a group of similarly affected individuals with epilepsy (see Chapter 15) [10, 30]. Without any type of intervention, the patient often becomes unassertive and isolated, losing interest in work, social activities, and family life [30].

One of the highest priorities after epilepsy develops is getting the patient back to work. This should be done even before seizure control is complete [8]. If seizures are frequent, this may not be feasible, but inactivity is too demoralizing to be encouraged. Unfortunately, many patients insist that seizure activity is the principal reason for their unemployment. Seventy percent of patients with epilepsy who do not work have more than one seizure every 6 months, and most have more than one seizure monthly [10]. Of those who are able to keep their jobs, only approximately one-half have seizures more than once per month.

What is cause and what is effect are much less definite than these statistics would suggest. That someone is working has an obvious, but unexplained, effect on seizure frequency: Patients with steady work exhibit fewer problems with seizure control than those who are unemployed [8]. The outcome after rehabilitation of any sort is better in younger adults than in older adults, a finding that is not surprising for this or any other medical condition [8]. An observation that is not so easily anticipated is that patients who receive welfare or other types of social assistance at the time a rehabilitative program is begun are much less likely ever to return to work than people with epilepsy who are still dependent on generating an income [10].

Mortality

The statistics on mortality of people with epilepsy suggest that there is an increased incidence of early death in this population, but the premature deaths usually are not caused by the epilepsy (Table 7–2) [31, 32]. The ratio of observed to expected deaths for individuals with epilepsy is 2.3:1 [31]. This mortality is inflated by including patients with epilepsy symptomatic of brain tumors, severe head trauma, congenital malformations, and strokes. If all patients with symptomatic epilepsy are excluded from the statistics, the mortality for the remaining individuals with idiopathic epilepsy is close to that of the general population [31]. There is little, if any, increased mortality among individuals with idiopathic generalized absence seizures, complex partial seizures, or rolandic epilepsy, especially if seizures first appeared in adolescence, seizure control is easily achieved, and the patient is female [31]. As with any condition that increases the risk of accidental injury, the observed increases in mortality are related to the severity of the disorder [32].

There are periods after the appearance of the epilepsy during which mortality is elevated. These include the first 2 years after an individual has his first seizure. Even if only one seizure is ever observed, mortality is more than twice that expected [31]. This early exacerbation of mortality is simply a reflection of the lethal character of some conditions that may cause seizures. Individuals who experience only one seizure have a normal mortality if they survive these first 2 years. Much more difficult to explain is a transient increase in the mortality 20 to 29 years after the initial diagnosis of the seizure disorder [31]. Also unexplained by current views on epilepsy is the lower long-term mortality for women, which is 1.6 over the course of 30 years, as compared to that for men, which is approximately 2.1 times the normal rate [31].

Certain types of epilepsy also have a poor prognosis. Myoclonic epilepsies, other than benign juvenile myoclonic epilepsy (see Chapter 2), are associated with a fourfold increase in mortality during the first year after the appearance of seizures [31]. Generalized tonic-clonic seizures are associated with a three-and-one-half-fold increase in mortality during the first year after seizure onset.

Table 7–2.
Factors Minimizing Mortality

Idiopathic seizures
Generalized absence, complex partial, or rolandic epilepsy
Easily achieved seizure control
Female sex
Onset of seizures in adolescence

Excluding obvious intracranial causes of seizure activity and early death, such as meningitis, brain tumors, and strokes, there are no natural causes of death that are common in the epileptic population but uncommon in the general population. Accidents, atherosclerotic vascular disease, and cancer are the commonest causes of death in patients with idiopathic epilepsy [33]. The one potentially lethal epileptic condition, status epilepticus, usually is not lethal if medical attention and effective antiepileptic treatment are obtained soon after its appearance.

Suicide and accidents are disturbingly common causes of death in patients with epilepsy, but the way in which these relate to the seizure disorder is controversial (see Chapter 13) [32–34]. Accidents cause 5 to 16 percent of the deaths in individuals with epilepsy, and an inordinately common accident is drowning [4, 32]. There is no evidence that antiepileptic medications play a role in the increased incidence of accidents [32]. Even though the incidence of suicide and accidents is increased, these do not contribute substantially to the mortality for the population with idiopathic seizures.

Unexplained death, in which the patient is found dead for no apparent reason and with no fatal lesions revealed by autopsy, has received relatively little attention, although it accounts for 5 to 30 percent of deaths in patients with epilepsy [35]. Most of these patients are found dead in bed or in other circumstances not suggestive of any protracted agonal problems. Sudden unexpected death occurs in approximately 1 of 1,100 individuals with epilepsy annually. Men are victims twice as often as women, and the seizure type generally associated with sudden unexplained death is generalized tonic-clonic epilepsy [35]. The victims usually are fairly young, the mean age at death being 27.6 years. However, there is a high incidence of alcoholism and a past history of head trauma among the victims. Frontal and temporal lobe contrecoup contusions are the commonest brain injuries found at autopsy [35].

Probably more important than any other factor in these unexplained deaths is the consistently inadequate antiepileptic treatment evident in the affected patients. At autopsy, 36 percent of sudden unexplained death victims have no antiepileptic drugs in their blood, and 68 percent have subtherapeutic levels [35]. Although this is speculation, it is likely that these patients died of cardiac arrhythmias induced by massive sympathetic discharges during a seizure. That the victims did not have effective anticonvulsant drug levels in most instances suggests that many of these unexplained deaths might be avoided with better antiepileptic drug compliance.

REFERENCES

1. Okuma, T., Kumashiro, H. Natural history and prognosis of epilepsy: report of a multi-institutional study in Japan. *Epilepsia* 22:35–53, 1981.
2. Lechtenberg, R. *Epilepsy and The Family.* Cambridge, Mass.: Harvard University Press, 1984.

3. Burden, G. Social aspects. In Reynolds, E.H., Trimble, M.R. (eds.), *Epilepsy and Psychiatry.* New York: Churchill Livingstone, 1981, p. 296–305.

4. Theodore, W.H., Schulman, E.A., Porter, R.J. Intractable seizures: long-term follow-up after prolonged inpatient treatment in an epilepsy unit. *Epilepsia* 24(3):336–343, 1983.

5. Reder, A.T., Wright, F.S. Epilepsy evoked by eating: the role of peripheral input. *Neurology* (N.Y.) 32(9):1065–1069, 1982.

6. Feldman, R.G., Paul, N.L. Identity of emotional triggers in epilepsy. *J. Nerv. Ment. Dis.* 162(5):345–353, 1976.

7. Mailick, M. The impact of severe illness on the individual and family: an overview. *Soc. Work Health Care* 5(2):117–128, 1979.

8. Schwartz, R.P. Epilepsy employment: a historical perspective. In The Commission for the Control of Epilepsy and its Consequences, *Plan for Nationwide Action on Epilepsy, Vol. 2.* Washington, D.C.: U.S. Department of Health, Education and Welfare, 1977, pp. 491–546.

9. Rodin, E.A. *The Prognosis of Patients with Epilepsy.* Springfield, Ill.: Charles C Thomas, 1968, p. 455.

10. Pigott, R.A. Evaluation of a Service Program focused on Vocational Rehabilitation as Prototype for an Urban Voluntary Epilepsy Agency. Boston: Epilepsy Society of Massachusetts, 1969, p. 124.

11. Bracht, N.F. The social nature of chronic disease and disability. *Soc. Work Health Care* 5(2):129–144, 1979.

12. Fraser, R.T., Clemmons, D., Trejo, W., Temkin, N.R. Program evaluation in epilepsy rehabilitation. *Epilepsia* 24(6):734–736, 1983.

13. Jerath, B.K., Kimbell, B.A. Hospitalization rates for epilepsy in the United States, 1973–1976. *Epilepsia* 22:55–64, 1981.

14. Bursten, B. Family dynamics, the sick role, and medical hospital admissions. *Fam. Process* 4(2):206–216, 1965.

15. Loiseau, P., Strube, E., Broustet, D., et al. Learning impairment in epileptic patients. *Epilepsia* 24(2):183–192, 1983.

16. Blumer, D. Temporal lobe epilepsy and its psychiatric significance. In Benson, D.F., Blumer D., (eds.), *Psychiatric Aspects of Neurologic Disease.* New York: Grune & Stratton, 1975, p. 171.

17. Masters, W.H., Johnson, V.E. *Human Sexual Response.* Boston: Little, Brown and Company, 1980.

18. Mohan, K.J., Salo, M.W., Nagaswani, S. A case of limbic system dysfunction with hypersexuality and fugue state. *Dis. Nerv. Syst.* 36:621, 1975.

19. Waxman, S.G., Geschwind, N. Hypergraphia in temporal lobe epilepsy. *Neurology* (N.Y.) 24:629, 1974.

20. Lindsay, J., Ounsted, C., Richards, P. Long-term outcome in children with temporal lobe seizures: II. Marriage, parenthood and sexual indifference. *Dev. Med. Child Neurol.* 21:433–440, 1979.

21. Remillard, G.M., Andermann, F., Testa, G.F., et al. Sexual ictal manifestations predominate in women with temporal lobe epilepsy: A finding suggesting sexual dimorphism in the human brain. *Neurology* (N.Y.) 33(3):323–330, 1983.

22. Kolarsky, A., Freund, K., Mochek, J., Polak, O. Male sexual deviation. Association with early temporal lobe damage. *Arch. Gen. Psychiatry* 17:735–743, 1967.

23. Taylor, D.C. Sexual behavior and temporal lobe epilepsy. *Arch. Neurol.* 21:510, 1969.

24. Waxman, S.G., Geschwind, N. The interictal behavior syndrome of temporal lobe epilepsy. *Arch. Gen. Psychiatry* 32:1580–1586, 1975.

25. Ellenberg, M. Sexual function in diabetic patients. *Ann. Intern. Med.* 92 (part 2):331, 1980.

26. Low, P.A., Walsh, J.C., Huang, C.Y., et al.   The sympathetic nervous system in diabetic neuropathy. *Brain* 98:341, 1975.
27. Hunter, R., Logue, V., McMenimy, W.H.   Temporal lobe epilepsy supervening on long-standing transvestism and fetishism. *Epilepsia* 4:60–65, 1973.
28. Currier, R.D., Little, S.C., Suess, J.F., Andy, O.J.   Sexual seizures. *Arch. Neurol.* 25:260–264, 1971.
29. Berg, B.O.   Prognosis of childhood epilepsy—another look. *N. Engl. J. Med.* 306(14):861–862, 1982.
30. Lessman, S.E., Mollick, L.R.   Group treatment of epileptics. *Health Soc. Work* 3(3):106–121, 1978.
31. Hauser, W.A., Annegers, J.F., Elveback, L.R.   Mortality in patients with epilepsy. *Epilepsia* 21:399–412, 1980.
32. Woodbury, L.A.   Shortening of the lifespan and mortality of patients with epilepsy. In The Commission for the Control of Epilepsy and Its Consequences, *Plan for Nationwide Action on Epilepsy*, vol 4. Washington, D.C.: U.S. Department of Health, Education and Welfare, 1978.
33. Barraclough, B.   Suicide and epilepsy. In Reynolds, E.H., Trimble, M.R. (eds.), *Epilepsy and Psychiatry.* New York: Churchill Livingstone, 1981, pp. 72–76.
34. Zielinski, J.J.   Epilepsy and mortality rate and cause of death. *Epilepsia* 16:191–201, 1974.
35. Leestma, J.A., Kalelkar, M.B., Teas, S.S., et al.   Sudden death associated with seizures: analysis of 66 cases. *Epilepsia* 25(1):84–88, 1984.

8. Reproduction and Birth Defects

Certain problems more common in patients with epilepsy than in the general population, such as mental retardation and other psychomotor handicaps, reduce the probability that some patients will reproduce, but even those unburdened by such obvious limitations exhibit lower than normal rates of marriage and child fostering. With advances in seizure control, this discrepancy between epileptic and normal populations is becoming less pronounced, but it is still present [1]. Marriage and fertility rates have increased substantially over the past generation for women with epilepsy, but not for men with epilepsy [1]. This is not reasonably ascribed to the patient's concerns with child fostering, since it is the woman who routinely has more concerns in this area. If a couple in which at least one partner is epileptic decides to have children, the epilepsy must be considered in the management of the pregnancy and observation of the newborn.

MARRIAGE RATES

Although patients obviously can have children without marrying, the documentable rate of reproduction in epileptic individuals is closely tied to the rate of marriage. Many patients with epilepsy never marry or have children. This is especially true for men: Approximately 70 percent of all men and women in the general population marry, whereas only 56 percent of epileptic men and 69 percent of epileptic women ever marry [2]. That marriage is less common in epileptic men than in the general population can be at least partly ascribed to their lack of sexual interest (see Chapter 7). That marriage rates are affected primarily for epileptic men rather than women may reflect a significant difference in social attitudes toward men with epilepsy, as opposed to those toward women, or it may indicate that subtle psychological effects of long-term epilepsy have different consequences for men and women [2]. An important social consideration is that men with seizures are considered less reliable providers than men without seizures, a fact that will influence marriage rates in societies where the man is expected to provide most of the financial support for the family.

The patient's age when the epilepsy first develops clearly plays a role in determining the likelihood of marriage for both men and women [1]. If the first seizure experienced by an individual occurs after the age of 20 years, that person is as likely to marry as any member of the general population [1]. Unfortunately, by 20 years of age, 75 percent of the people who will develop epilepsy in their lifetimes have already done so [1]. If the patient developed epilepsy during childhood but his seizures were fully controlled by the time he was 12 years old, he is as likely to marry as anyone in the general population [3]. Marriages involving men with poorly controlled epilepsy since childhood usually end in early separation or divorce [3].

Aside from a lack of interest and social prejudice, additional factors that decrease the marriage rate for men with epilepsy may include a characteristic lack of initiative and assertiveness. Even those epileptic men with some interest in marrying and having a family are less likely to propose marriage than non-epileptic men. Obviously, these characteristics are not found only in men with epilepsy: They are simply more prevalent in the epileptic population than in the population at large.

REPRODUCTIVE RATES

Epileptic women who marry have only 69 percent of the live-born children expected for married women in the general population, whereas those relatively few epileptic men who marry have as many children in their families as the average married man [1]. Statistics for children born out of wedlock to these individuals are not available, but it appears that whether or not they are married, reproductive rates are depressed for epileptic men and women who can be sexually active. The reproductive rate is affected by several different factors including the type of epilepsy exhibited by the patient. Married women with complex partial seizures have an average of 1.64 children each, whereas married men with this type of seizure disorder have an average of 0.54 children each [3].

Effect of Antiepileptics on Fertility

Antiepileptic drugs do not interfere with fertility. In fact, women taking both hormonal contraceptive pills and antiepileptics may have unwanted fertility. Some antiepileptic drugs, including phenytoin, interfere with the levels of hormones maintained by the contraceptive pill, and the lowered hormone levels increase the risk of pregnancy. An obvious solution is to administer contraceptive pills with higher hormone contents, but risks associated with these higher estrogen or progesterone preparations may not justify their use in the woman with epilepsy. An alternative contraceptive, such as an intrauterine device or cervical cap, should be considered. Gynecologic studies to determine whether ovulation is occurring may show that the contraceptive pill is not being effective, but failure to detect ovulation does not establish the reliability of the contraceptive pill.

Risk of Miscarriage

The smaller number of living children born to epileptic women is not a result of a higher than normal rate of miscarriage in these women on antiepileptic drugs. Women with epilepsy have the same rate of spontaneous abortion as nonepileptic women (14 percent) [1]. The difference in the average number of children per family seems to be primarily from a lower rate of conception: Women with epilepsy do not become pregnant as often during their marriages as women without epilepsy. There is also a slightly higher rate of stillbirths in women with epilepsy, and this is unrelated to whether they take medication [4].

PREGNANCY AND EPILEPSY

Of all the women who become pregnant, at least 2.1 percent have had a seizure at some time in their lives or have a seizure during the pregnancy [4]. Approximately 4.5 of every 1,000 women who become pregnant have had a seizure within 5 years of the pregnancy and an additional 4.4 of every 1,000 have at least one seizure during the pregnancy that is not related to eclampsia [4]. These women do not necessarily have epilepsy, since, in many cases, the seizure occurs only once and does not represent a persistent neurologic problem. However, 1 to 8 percent of the women who are pregnant at any one time have had more than one seizure before they became pregnant [5].

The combination of a history of seizures and a diagnosis of pregnancy presents several problems and concerns for the affected woman. That a seizure has occurred at some time in her past raises the possibility that the stress of pregnancy will precipitate more seizures. If the patient is taking an antiepileptic drug, she must deal with changes in the way the medication is metabolized during the pregnancy, as well as with the effects of the medication on the fetus. If she is not being medicated, she may have increased seizure activity and cause injuries to the fetus during the attacks. Of course, even women who have never had seizures may develop them during pregnancy. These women should be started on antiepileptic drugs if the seizures are idiopathic or persistent, but whether such therapy should be continued at the end of the pregnancy must be decided on an individual basis.

Toxic Complications of Antiepileptic Drugs

Most antiepileptic drugs pose no special problems for the mother or the fetus as long as serum drug levels are maintained below the toxic range. One notable exception is phenytoin. Phenytoin lowers serum folate and interferes with vitamin K metabolism [6, 7]. If vitamin K levels are chronically low, bleeding disorders theoretically could develop in both the mother and the newborn. Actual bleeding disorders in such circumstances have not been documented, but precautions should be taken nonetheless. The possibility of a phenytoin-associated bleeding disorder can be minimized by giving supplementary vitamin K to the patient during the last few months of her pregnancy and by injecting vitamin K into the child at or shortly after birth [6].

Other adverse effects of antiepileptic medications must be watched for during the pregnancy, even if they never occurred before the woman became pregnant. Changes in hormone levels and organ sensitivities to a variety of drugs may precipitate hepatic, renal, or dermatologic problems at drug levels that were previously innocuous. Fortunately, these effects are very unlikely to occur, and drug changes based on a newly acquired intolerance rarely are needed at any time during the pregnancy.

Effects of Pregnancy on Antiepileptics

Pregnancy affects antiepileptic drugs in several ways. It often reduces the absorption of the drug, increases the rate of turnover, and presents a greater volume in which the drug must be distributed [4]. Serum anticonvulsant levels routinely fall as the pregnancy progresses, and the patient becomes more vulnerable to seizure activity. The rate at which the drug level falls is unpredictable and must be monitored every 3 to 6 weeks. A therapeutic drug level can be maintained by adjusting the dose of medication when necessary.

The required amount of medication generally increases most substantially during the second and third trimester of the pregnancy, whereas any birth defects that might be induced by the antiepileptic drug are most likely to develop during the first trimester of pregnancy. Therefore, concern for the fetus is no reason to allow the mother's serum drug levels to fall later in the pregnancy. In fact, ineffective serum drug levels are an unwise approach to protecting the fetus at any time during the pregnancy and place the mother in an unacceptably dangerous position. Any changes in a patient's antiepileptic drug regimen that are intended to protect the fetus should be completed before the patient becomes pregnant.

Immediately after the completion or termination of the pregnancy, the woman's required dose of antiepileptic usually falls. To avoid a toxic reaction at this point, the amount of medication given must be reduced, again with the rate of change in medication dictated by changes in serum levels of the drug.

Effects of Seizures on the Fetus

Most women with epilepsy or a history of seizures have normal children. However, if seizures occur during the pregnancy, the fetus is at risk along with the patient. Most seizures will not cause permanent damage to either the mother or the fetus, but a fall suffered during a tonic-clonic seizure may be as damaging to the fetus as it is to the mother (or more so). If there are risks to the fetus from the metabolic changes occurring during a seizure, they are difficult to document.

The analysis of the effect of seizures alone on a pregnancy is complicated by the confounding effect of a history of anticonvulsant medication use. Most women who experience seizures take antiepileptic drugs during the pregnancy, and virtually all except those whose seizures first develop during the pregnancy have taken anticonvulsants at some time prior to the pregnancy [5]. Even if the patient does not take medication during the pregnancy, earlier exposure to drugs may be responsible for problems appearing in the fetus. This remote effect of anticonvulsants is extremely unlikely, but it makes difficult the evaluation of any complications appearing during pregnancy.

Effects of Pregnancy on Epilepsy

Epilepsy is not usually affected substantially by pregnancy if the woman has routine medical and neurologic follow-up [8]. Medical follow-up may involve little more than routine checkups by an obstetrician. The neurologic follow-up must involve monthly checks of antiepileptic drug levels in serum. In at least half of the epileptic women whose pregnancies go to term, there is no change in the level of seizure control during the pregnancy (Table 8–1) [8]. In approximately 37 percent, seizure frequency is increased, and 13 percent will have less frequent seizures [8].

When seizure frequency increases, the cause is poor drug compliance or obvious sleep deprivation in 68 percent of epileptic women [8]. The poor compliance often occurs because the expectant mother is concerned about the effect of the antiepileptic medication on the fetus. Some physicians even encourage their patients to decrease the dose of medication taken during the

Table 8–1.
Causes of Epilepsy During Pregnancy

For woman known to have epilepsy
Poor drug compliance
Sleep deprivation
Altered antiepileptic drug metabolism

For woman without previous epilepsy
Occult seizure disorder
Eclampsia
Subarachnoid hemorrhage
Stroke

---

first few months of pregnancy, because they, too, believe that the drugs pose an unacceptable risk for the fetus. That any adverse effects of the antiepileptics on the fetus are dose-related has not been established, but there is some evidence that the risk of malformation is correlated, to some extent, with the maternal levels of phenytoin or phenobarbital if these are the principal anticonvulsants used [7, 8]. The importance of the drug serum level in inducing malformations and the role played by depression of serum folate by these drugs are unknown, but it is clear that inadequate maternal drug serum levels are dangerous for the mother [7].

Approximately 47 percent of the epileptic women with increased seizure frequency during pregnancy will also prove to have less than therapeutic levels of anticonvulsants in their serum [8]. When seizures decrease in frequency, it is usually because the woman is under closer supervision. The antiepileptic drug level is more likely to be checked and compliance improves.

Onset of Epilepsy During Pregnancy

Seizures sometimes occur for the first time, or recur after years of apparent remission, during pregnancy. When seizures occur along with hypertension and changes in renal function, the woman has eclampsia or toxemia of pregnancy. When the seizures occur in an otherwise uncomplicated pregnancy, they may be evidence of a fairly low seizure threshold that is exceeded because of the stress of pregnancy. Although pregnancy may not cause extraordinary stress for most women, it does involve dramatic hormonal changes in all women. These hormonal changes may contribute to the development of epilepsy, but the epilepsy may remit when the pregnancy ends.

A more sinister possibility is that the patient has an occult brain lesion which is responsible for the seizures but that the lesion, whether a tumor, hamartoma, or other structural problem, is not adequately irritating to be symptomatic without the provocative influence of the pregnancy. An inordinately large proportion of women who have their first seizures during pregnancy will have evidence of mental retardation on formal neuropsychological testing [4]. Black women often prove to have sickle cell disease [4]. In both situations, the seizure probably is evidence of previously unsuspected brain damage from a developmental problem or a minor stroke.

Seizures occurring during labor are more worrisome than those occurring during the pregnancy, because the exertion and agitation typical of labor may precipitate bleeding from occult aneurysms or arteriovenous malformations. A woman without these vascular abnormalities is not at risk, but which women have the faulty vessels will not be apparent until after the subarachnoid or intracerebral hemorrhage has occurred.

Seizures occurring during the pregnancy may be no more than the recurrence of a long-standing but unrecognized problem. Young women developing seizures while pregnant may not recall seizures that they suffered in infancy.

Because there are so many possible causes of seizures during pregnancy, treatment is not a simple matter. Anticonvulsants should be given to the pregnant woman with seizures as soon as the physician is confident that there is no reversible metabolic or infectious basis for the seizure. If an obvious metabolic problem, such as hypocalcemia or hyponatremia, is found, that problem should be corrected before antiepileptic drugs are begun. If the patient has a fever and stiff neck, meningitis or meningoencephalitis should be sought with examination of the cerebrospinal fluid. If the seizures are not symptomatic of these usually obvious problems, anticonvulsants should be given until the cause of the seizures can be established.

The physician responsible for the woman with new seizures should be reluctant to use any investigative techniques that would be hazardous for the fetus, but the mother's health has priority. If it is feasible, studies requiring ionizing radiation, such as computed tomography, or other modalities potentially damaging to the fetus should be delayed until the pregnancy is completed. This is not a consideration if an induced abortion is planned. The scatter of radiation with a computed tomogram of the head is negligible, but the woman subjected to this type of procedure who subsequently has a deformed baby may reject assurances that the ionizing radiation played no role in the bad outcome. A lumbar puncture to check the cerebrospinal fluid for blood or infection poses no threat to the fetus and should not be delayed if it is likely to help in the investigation of the seizures. Ultrasonic studies of the brain are also safe and may provide evidence of a large intracranial mass.

Treatment of Seizures Occurring with Pregnancy

The selection of an antiepileptic drug to suppress seizures that appear during pregnancy will depend on the type of seizure occurring and the stage of pregnancy in which it occurs. If the problem appears during the first trimester, anticonvulsants likely to cause birth defects should be avoided, even though the risks are small. This means that of the commonly used drugs, phenytoin, primidone, and phenobarbital are inadvisable early in the pregnancy, unless the patient was taking these medications before she became pregnant.

Pregnancy is the wrong time to introduce new antiepileptic regimens. Drug changes are particularly unwise early in pregnancy, because they expose the patient to the risks of drug withdrawal and may leave her on a new drug that provides inadequate protection from seizures. Many women do not realize they are pregnant until late in their first trimester, by which time the antiepileptics may have already caused problems for the fetus. This means that the possibility of a future pregnancy should play a role in determining which medication will be prescribed for a young woman. Drugs that carry excessively high risks of fetal malformation, such as trimethadione, should be scrupulously avoided.

Although no antiepileptic drug is unequivocally free of adverse effects on the embryo, some have less well documented teratogenicity than others. Of the commonly used drugs, carbamazepine and valproic acid currently appear to carry the lowest risk. The woman who develops seizures early in pregnancy and requires anticonvulsant treatment should be started on one of these two drugs if her seizure type is one on which these drugs exhibit some effectiveness.

If seizures occur during labor, an oral anticonvulsant may be impractical. Although intravenous medication will assure good seizure control in a very short period of time, this approach may pose unnecessary complications for the anesthesiologist. Intramuscular medication usually is adequate to get the patient through labor with no more seizures and little sedation of the neonate. Phenobarbital is a good drug to use in such situations, because effective levels can be achieved quickly and sustained for several hours after a single injection of 100 to 300 mg.

If the labor is not likely to be protracted, diazepam may provide equally good protection, but it is best administered intravenously in 5- to 10-mg boluses, which may sedate the newborn. Any antiepileptic given near the time of delivery must be viewed as a potential problem for the newborn as well as the mother, but the risks are minimal if the obstetrician and anesthesiologist are aware of the medications given and are prepared to manage a sedated infant. When seizures are more difficult to suppress and the mother must be heavily sedated with antiepileptics, a neonatologist should be involved in the delivery (whenever that is practical) to deal with problems faced by the newborn.

Birth Defects in Offspring of Epileptic Women

Whether or not a woman who has had seizures takes antiepileptic medication, the incidence of stillbirths, microcephaly, mental retardation, and nonfebrile seizures in her children will be greater than that in the general population of children born to women who have never had seizures [4]. Offspring of women with noneclamptic seizures are in some way abnormal at 1 year of age four

Table 8–2.
Birth Defects in Offspring of Women on Antiepileptic Drugs

Type of Defect	Percentage of All Birth Defects
Skeletal abnormalities (e.g., limb hypoplasia, hip dislocations)	22.7%
Cardiovascular abnormalities Ventricular septal defects (5.3%)	17.7%
Facial anomalies Cleft lip or palate (16.2%)	17.2%
Gastrointestinal anomalies	9.7%
Genitourinary anomalies (e.g., hypospadias)	9.2%
Central nervous system defects (e.g., microcephaly)	7.8%

times as often as other children, even though they do not have an increased incidence of low birth weights, neonatal seizures, or death during the first year of life (Table 8–2) [4]. Stillbirths are especially common among women who have had at least one seizure during the pregnancy, but in most cases, the cause of the seizures seems to be the cause of the stillbirths [4]; the seizures themselves are not lethal for the fetus. Even when seizures have occurred as remotely as 1, 2, or even 5 years before the pregnancy, the incidence of stillbirths is twice that found in the general population [4].

Febrile seizures are four times greater than normal for the offspring of women who have had seizures within 5 years of the pregnancy, and these febrile seizures are followed by nonfebrile seizures eleven times the norm in the progeny of mothers with epilepsy or a history of a single seizure within 5 years of the pregnancy [4]. The children also have a higher incidence of retarded (below 70) intelligence quotients (I.Q.s). In fact, cerebral palsy, nonfebrile seizures, an I.Q. below 70, or a head circumference more than two standard deviations below the norm is twice as common in the offspring of women who have had seizures within 5 years of pregnancy and even more common if a seizure occurred during the pregnancy itself [4]. The mother's use or nonuse of antiepileptic drugs during or before the pregnancy does not affect these statistics [4].

Because of these and other observations, the fetal problems directly attributable to antiepileptic drugs are controversial. Contributing to the confusion is the limited opportunity to follow women with epilepsy who become pregnant and do not use antiepileptic drugs. Few of these control women have been studied, and most are younger than the general population of epileptic women completing pregnancies.

Even if it is assumed that the antiepileptic drug taken by the mother is the immediate cause of the child's birth defects, it is often impossible to relate specific defects to specific drugs, because many pregnant epileptic women are taking more than one drug or even more than one antiepileptic drug during the pregnancy. The possibility of complex drug interactions muddles the assessment of individual agents. Differences in the extent of follow-up and the criteria used for identifying malformations in the fetus or newborn also produce disagreements between different studies [5]. It can be said with confidence, however, that women with epilepsy have children with more birth defects than would be expected for comparable women in the general population, and epileptic women who require anticonvulsant drugs on a long-term basis have children with an even higher incidence of birth defects.

The rate of malformations in children of all women with epilepsy is approximately one and four-fifths times that observed in children of nonepileptic mothers [5]. Although some studies have shown no increased incidence of birth defects among children of epileptic mothers who have not been treated with anticonvulsants, this may have more to do with the type of patient that is left untreated than with the actual risk of malformations when a pregnant epileptic woman is not given antiepileptic drugs [5]. The woman not treated for seizures usually is younger, less severely impaired by seizures, and less frequently exhibits seizures than the woman who is on drugs [5]. Birth defects are increased whether or not the mother takes anticonvulsants during the pregnancy, but the rate of defects is five times as great in the woman who does take drugs [9]. The risk faced seems to vary with the drug taken, but many factors enter into determining which drug the woman is taking. The highest rate of fetal maldevelopment (12.7 percent) occurs in women on multiple anticonvulsants who have persistent seizures during their pregnancies despite this drug regimen [9].

Spectrum of Birth Defects

The variety of malformations that develop in children born to women on antiepileptic drugs is not substantially different from that observed in the general population [5]. The commonest malformations are cleft lip or palate, heart anomalies, and skeletal malformations [9]. Cleft lip is twelve times as common as in the general population, and heart anomalies are eighteen times as common [9]. Congenital hip dislocations are forty times as common as in the general population, but this is a relatively rare birth defect when compared to facial and heart anomalies [9].

All types of skeletal anomalies account for approximately 23 percent of the abnormalities occurring in these children, but many of them are too minor to be considered a true deformity [5]. Some of the more serious skeletal problems that occur include distal limb hypoplasia, clubfoot, and hip dislocations. The commonest anomalies that are defects by any criteria are those occurring in the cardiovascular system, and the most common of these are ventricular septal defects [5].

Cleft lip and palate occur almost as frequently (16 percent of observed anomalies) as the cardiovascular malformations [5]. Nervous system defects account for only 8 percent or so of the anomalies in these children, and both genitourinary and gastrointestinal anomalies occur more frequently than this [5]. Microcephaly, hypospadias, and diaphragmatic hernias are the commonest anomalies occurring in these systems.

Risk with Specific Drugs
The roles of genetic factors that contribute to the appearance of epilepsy and of antiepileptic drugs in causing birth defects are not yet well defined. Certain types of drugs seem to present a high risk for the fetus. Drugs in the oxazolidinedione family, such as trimethadione and paramethadione, are most unequivocally associated with a high incidence of developmental defects [5, 9]. Significant correlations have also been found between the ingestion of primidone, phenobarbital, and acetazolamide and an increased incidence of birth defects [9].

Phenytoin may cause craniofacial and skeletal anomalies in some infants exposed to the drug during fetal life, but this type of anomaly is fairly common in families of individuals with idiopathic epilepsy, regardless of the history of fetal drug exposure [5]. Studies on the effect of phenytoin on animal fetuses suggested that the increased incidence of cleft lip and palate in infants exposed to the drug was caused by the drug, but phenytoin is metabolized differently in different animals [5]. A syndrome called the *fetal hydantoin syndrome,* in which several malformations appear together in newborns exposed while in utero to phenytoin (diphenylhydantoin), has been recognized for many years, but its validity still is somewhat controversial [5, 10]. Some physicians believe that it is not clearly specific for phenytoin exposure or even for antiepileptic exposure (see Chapter 14). Little more than slow growth and development are evident in the majority of infants exposed to effective anticonvulsant levels of phenytoin during the early months of fetal development [11]. Serious malformations appear in approximately 10 percent of infants born to epileptic women taking phenytoin, but even twins exhibit different developmental patterns after exposure to the drug [11].

Carbamazepine and valproic acid produce no appreciable increase in the rate of birth defects, but the experience with valproic acid has been too limited to assume it will not cause problems in any fetuses [5, 9]. Valproic acid accumulates in fetal blood, a property not shared with phenytoin, primidone, phenobarbital, carbamazepine, or ethosuximide, and so fetal effects may be more dose-related than with other antiepileptic drugs [12]. Primidone and phenobarbital are associated with a slightly lower incidence of birth defects than phenytoin, but the pattern of defects is much the same.

Importance of Epilepsy in the Father

If the father has epilepsy because of a hereditary neurologic problem, such as tuberous sclerosis, the child is obviously at a greater risk of having birth defects than the child of parents with no hereditary disorders. Statistics on birth defects in the offspring of epileptic fathers may not accurately reflect more subtle effects of epilepsy or anticonvulsant treatment in the father, because the child's paternity cannot be established from questionnaires and population surveys alone. Some studies indicate that the children of epileptic men who have taken anticonvulsants have more malformations than the offspring of epileptic men never treated with anticonvulsants [13]. This does not mean, however, that the drugs necessarily caused damage to the sperm. It may simply indicate that men not treated for seizures are very different genetically from men who invariably require medication for the management of their seizures. It is very possible that sperm are damaged directly by the antiepileptic agents, but if such damage occurs, it must be at a relatively low frequency for obvious defects to have eluded detection for so long.

PUERPERAL SEIZURES

When seizures occur in the mother during the first few hours or days after the delivery, it is usually because of a lapse in medication. If the woman has no oral intake because of a cesarean section or complicated vaginal delivery, her antiepileptic drug level will fall steadily. The combination of stress, blood loss, and fatigue could easily precipitate a seizure even if the woman were well medicated, but with inadequate serum antiepileptic levels, she is at substantial risk of having seizures. This is avoided by providing either intramuscular or intravenous medication while the woman is unable to take her usual oral medications. Phenobarbital, 100 mg intramuscularly daily, or phenytoin, 300 mg intravenously (at no more than 50 mg/min) are the most readily available and reliable drugs appropriate during the period without oral intake.

Seizures appearing for the first time during the puerperium usually indicate a new central nervous system lesion. This may be a subarachnoid hemorrhage that was not evident during the delivery or an infection that developed as a complication of the delivery. Seizures are not usually the first sign of sepsis, but malaise and low-grade fever may be mistaken for unimportant signs of exhaustion and local trauma after a difficult delivery. With the appearance of seizures, a computed tomogram should be obtained immediately to check for an intracerebral hemorrhage, and a lumbar puncture should follow within minutes if the scan is negative. Pituitary infarction at the time of delivery may produce a life-threatening chemical meningitis that may respond to high-dose steroid treatment. If there appears to be a meningitis, intravenous antibiotic treatment must be started even before the organism is identified.

BREAST-FEEDING

Breast-feeding poses no threat to the infant born to an epileptic woman on therapeutic doses of antiepileptic medication, even if the nursing mother is taking more than one antiepileptic drug. Primidone, phenobarbital, ethosuximide, and carbamazepine are excreted in maternal milk in sufficient quantities to produce measurable levels in the nursing infants, but the serum concentrations in the infants seem to be inconsequential [12]. The amounts of valproic acid and phenytoin excreted in milk are unequivocally negligible [12]. Even if the nursing mother is on antiepileptic medication, development of the newborn should proceed at a normal pace if the infant is healthy. Any developmental delays should be investigated.

One problem that does arise with breast-feeding is that the epileptic woman often becomes sleep-deprived [8]. The demands imposed by the infant for attention at irregular intervals throughout the night can induce seizures in the nursing mother as she adopts the irregular schedule. Women with epilepsy and newborns should be encouraged to share responsibilities with other family members, at least at night, so that a relatively normal sleep pattern can be maintained. This may mean feeding the child with formula when nursing is inconvenient.

REFERENCES

1. Dansky, L.V., Andermann, E., Andermann, F. Marriage and fertility in epileptic patients. *Epilepsia* 21:261–271, 1980.
2. Tsuboi, T. Incidence of seizures among offspring of epileptic patients. In Janz, D., Dam, M., Richens, A., et al. (eds.), *Epilepsy, Pregnancy, and the Child.* New York: Raven Press, 1982, pp. 527–534.
3. Lindsay, J., Ounsted, C., Richards, P. Long-term outcome in children with temporal lobe seizures: II. Marriage, parenthood and sexual indifference. *Dev. Med. Child Neurol.* 21:433–440, 1979.
4. Nelson, K.B., Ellenberg, J.H. Maternal seizure disorder, outcome of pregnancy, and neurologic abnormalities in the children. *Neurology* (N.Y.) 32(11):1247–1254, 1982.
5. Bossi, L. Fetal effects of anticonvulsants. In Morselli, P.L., Pippenger, C.E., Penry, J.K. (eds.), *Antiepileptic Drug Therapy in Pediatrics.* New York: Raven Press, 1983, pp. 37–64.
6. Jennett, B. Epilepsy after head injury and craniotomy. In Godwin-Austen, R.B., Espir, M.L.E. (eds.), *Driving and Epilepsy.* Royal Society of Medicine International Congress and Symposium Series, no. 60. London: Academic Press, 1983, pp. 49–51.
7. Dansky, L., Andermann, E., Andermann, F., et al. Antiepileptic drug levels, folate, and birth defects: a prospective study. *Epilepsia* 24(4):520, 1983.
8. Schmidt, D., Canger, R., Avanzini, G., et al. Change of seizure frequency in pregnant epileptic women. *J. Neurol. Neurosurg. Psychiatry* 46:751–755, 1983.
9. Nakane, Y., Okuma, T., Takahashi, R., et al. Multi-institutional study on the teratogenicity and fetal toxicity of antiepileptic drugs: a report of a collaborative study group in Japan. *Epilepsia* 21:663–680, 1980.
10. Hanson, J.W., Smith, D.W. The fetal hydantoin syndrome. *J. Pediatr.* 87:285–290, 1975.
11. Phelan, M.C., Pellock, J.M., Nance, W.E. Discordant expression of fetal hydantoin syndrome in heteropaternal dizygotic twins. *N. Engl. J. Med.* 307:99–101, 1982.

12. Nau, H., Kuhnz, W., Rating, D., et al.   Anticonvulsants during pregnancy and the lactation period: pharmacokinetics and clinical studies. *Epilepsia* 24(2):253, 1983.
13. Meyer, J.G.   The teratological effects of anticonvulsants and the effect on pregnancy and birth. *Eur. Neurol.* 10:179–190, 1973.

9. Inheritance of Epilepsy

Some of the conditions that cause epilepsy are familial, and so epilepsy occasionally appears to be hereditary. However, to refer to it as a hereditary problem is misleading, since many patients with the neurologic diseases responsible for the familial patterns observed have no seizures. Those diseases that may give rise to epilepsy are transmitted as dominant, recessive, or X-linked traits [1]. Penetrance of the dominant and X-linked traits is variable [1]. Most of the autosomal recessive and X-linked disorders are enzyme defects, many of which have been characterized [2]. If the cause of the epilepsy is unknown, but there is a familial pattern to the occurrence of the seizure disorder, it is difficult to escape the view that the epilepsy is a hereditary problem. Keeping these qualifications in mind, it is still fair to say that most people with epilepsy will not transmit the disorder to their offspring.

Hereditary disorders causing epilepsy include congenital malformations of the brain, disorders of metabolism, and recurrent tumor formation. An adult without epilepsy may have a hereditary neurologic disorder that causes epilepsy in his or her children. In some cases, the hereditary defect is nothing more than a recurrent abnormality in electroencephalographic activity. Presumably, this brain wave abnormality is from a metabolic or organizational problem in the brain, but the physiologic basis for the defect is not apparent. This does not mean that the risk of developing epilepsy is substantial if a parent or grandparent has or had epilepsy. Overall, the risk that epilepsy will appear in a child with an affected relative is small, simply because many epilepsies develop secondary to head injuries, central nervous system infections, and strokes.

RISK OF INHERITANCE

The risk that a child with one affected parent will develop epilepsy is five times that of an individual in the general population, but that still places the risk at only 2 to 5 children of 100 with epileptic parents (Table 9–1) [1, 3]. With dominantly inherited disorders, the risk that a child will develop the epilepsy exhibited by an affected parent may be as high as 50 percent [1]. In twins, if one develops epilepsy, there is an increased risk that the other will also; this risk ranges from 5 to 20 percent for fraternal twins to 40 to 90 percent for identical twins [1].

Considering the cause of the epilepsy, the parent affected by the seizure disorder, and the type of seizure disorder in the parent, one finds that a child is at highest risk of developing epilepsy if the affected parent is the mother and if this parent has idiopathic generalized seizures with no auras [3, 4]. Regardless of which parent has the epilepsy, sons are more likely to develop the problem than daughters [3]. The incidence of seizures in the offspring of an epileptic parent may be as high as 12 percent, but this statistic includes children who have only one observed seizure in their childhood and who may never develop epilepsy [4]. Unequivocal epilepsy will develop in 2.9 percent of the sons and 2.3 percent of the daughters of epileptic women, and in 1.1 percent of the sons and 0.6 percent of the daughters of epileptic men [4].

The reasons that children of an epileptic woman are more likely to develop the problem than children of an epileptic man are unknown. Part of the statistical difference may be an artifact of mistaken identity: The wrong man is more likely than the wrong woman to be identified as the parent. An alternative explanation is that birth complications play a part in the development of some seizure disorders, and women with epilepsy are more likely to have complicated gestations and deliveries than women without epilepsy [3].

Occasionally, the first individual recognized to have seizures is the child. Other relatives with so-called drop attacks, episodic confusion, blackouts, and

Table 9–1.
Factors Associated With an Increased Risk of Inheriting Epilepsy

Mother has seizures
Offspring at risk is male
Parent has idiopathic generalized seizures
Parent's seizures lack an aura
Several members of the family have epilepsy
Relatives have metabolic disease knows to cause epilepsy

transient memory lapses will be recognized as having epilepsy only after the child's seizures are diagnosed. If a child has epilepsy, the prevalence of epilepsy in his parents may be as high as 14 percent; in his siblings, as high as 3 percent; in distant relatives, as high as 2.8 percent [4].

CHARACTERISTICS OF THE HEREDITARY DISORDER

In children who develop seizures on a hereditary basis that are unrelated to a lethal metabolic problem, the epilepsy follows a fairly consistent pattern. If seizures are going to develop, they usually appear between 5 and 19 years of age [4]. The type of epilepsy developing is generally that observed in the parent, but the age of onset for the child may be slightly earlier than that seen in the parent. A notable exception to both of these rules occurs if the parent has focal motor or focal sensory epilepsy. Children of parents with focal epilepsies often develop generalized epilepsy, and that epilepsy routinely begins by 2 years of age if it is ever going to develop [3].

In some families, the inheritance of epilepsy is less apparent than the inheritance of a low seizure threshold in particular settings. The most obvious example of this is with complex partial seizures. Most of the known causes of complex partial seizures are not hereditary, but 2.6 percent of the relatives of patients with this type of epilepsy will themselves have some form of epilepsy, though not necessarily the complex partial type [5]. Lowered resistance to seizure activity of several types seems to be inherited in these families.

COMMONLY INHERITED SEIZURE TYPES

Some seizure disorders have well-defined hereditary patterns (Table 9–2). The classic form of generalized absence epilepsy, which has a characteristic three-per-second spike-and-wave pattern, is one of the most commonly occurring types of hereditary epilepsy. This typical petit mal is transmitted in a dominant pattern, but individuals with the genetic material that can cause these seizures do not necessarily have clinical seizures [1, 6]. Adults who carry the gene or genes responsible for the disorder may exhibit three-per-second spike-and-slow wave patterns on their electroencephalograms even if they

Table 9–2.
Seizure Disorders With Familial Patterns

Febrile seizures
Generalized absence seizures
Idiopathic complex partial epilepsy
Benign focal epilepsy of childhood
Benign juvenile myoclonic epilepsy
Myoclonic photosensitive epilepsy

do not experience seizures [1, 6]. If absence seizures are going to develop in a child as part of a hereditary disorder, they usually appear between 5 and 9 years of age [6]. If the very young child has the typical three-per-second spike-and-wave pattern of generalized absence epilepsy but no apparent seizures, the seizures will develop before adolescence in 25 percent of cases [1]. Even if the child never develops epilepsy, 35 percent of his offspring will also exhibit this electroencephalographic pattern, at least during childhood [1].

Rolandic epilepsy is also dominantly inherited with variable penetrance [6]. Approximately one-third of the siblings of children with this benign focal epilepsy of childhood exhibit brain wave changes, even if they have no seizures [7]. Presumably, there is a transient metabolic or membrane defect transmitted in these families, but the nature of the defect has never been determined.

Complex partial epilepsy appears more often in the immediate family of an individual with this type of seizure disorder than is expected in the general population. The siblings and children of patients with idiopathic complex partial seizures have electroencephalographic patterns suggestive of seizure activity in 20 percent of cases, even when no seizures are observed in these relatives [7]. These members of the immediate family have a 7 percent risk of suffering one or more seizures and a 4 percent risk of developing a chronic seizure disorder [7].

Simple febrile seizures exhibit a strong familial pattern, but they are not accurately described as a form of epilepsy. The child with simple febrile seizures often has only one or two in his lifetime and never requires medication. The conditions needed to provoke the seizures are also very well defined. Seizures invariably occur when the child is between 6 months and 4 years of age and only at the peak of a rapidly rising temperature spike (see Chapter 5) [6]. The tendency to have these seizures appears to be transmitted in a dominant manner with variable penetrance [6].

Several other less common seizure disorders also exhibit hereditary patterns, but in these, the epilepsy can often be traced to a hereditary metabolic disorder. Myoclonic photosensitive epilepsy is one such seizure disorder. This is a dominantly inherited problem in which flashes of light will precipitate seizures with prominent limb or truncal jerking movements [6]. The patient usually has a brief absence or trance as part of the seizure. On the electroencephalogram, this may look very much like generalized absence epilepsy. A child may induce his own attacks by waving his hands in front of his face or by watching a flickering television screen [6]. This seizure disorder actually may be the initial sign of a storage disease, such as Lafora body disease, which causes central nervous system damage and produces a myoclonic epilepsy [6].

Benign juvenile myoclonic epilepsy is much more common than myoclonic photosensitive epilepsy, but the two share some features, including a sensitivity to photic stimulation and a familial pattern of transmission [8]. The precise pattern of inheritance for benign juvenile myoclinic epilepsy is unknown [8].

Hereditary Nervous System Diseases

Epilepsy is a symptom of several hereditary nervous system disorders that damage or irritate the cerebral cortex [2]. It is rarely an expression of a disease that disturbs the subcortical white matter. The seizure disorder usually is not the only symptom of the hereditary disease, but it is very often the initial or most prominent sign of brain damage. Most hereditary nervous system disorders are associated with systemic effects of the genetic disease. The skin is an especially common site for signs outside the central nervous system. The child with a facial port-wine spot may have vascular abnormalities overlying the brain that are characteristic of Sturge-Weber syndrome. Other central nervous system disorders that cause epilepsy and have obvious skin manifestations include tuberous sclerosis and neurofibromatosis. Inborn errors of metabolism that cause epilepsy in the first days or months of life usually are lethal [1].

Disorders Apparent in Infancy

Most of the metabolic problems causing seizures in neonates and infants also cause mental retardation. Although the chemical bases for several of these disorders have been identified, treatment is available for only a few.

Phenylketonuria is one of the more common causes of seizures and mental retardation in infants, and it is one of the most treatable [1]. Newborn blood can be checked for abnormal handling of phenylalanine, and if the tests indicate phenylketonuria, a diet deficient in phenylalanine may suffice to avoid significant retardation and epilepsy [1]. Women with this disorder should be discouraged from having children, because their offspring usually develop intellectual problems and seizures, even though these children do not have phenylketonuria [1]. The mother with phenylketonuria may have in her blood during the pregnancy levels of phenylalanine that she can tolerate well but that are toxic to the nervous system of the fetus.

A less common, but equally treatable, cause of seizures in newborns is pyridoxine dependency. Infants with this disorder require excessively high levels of this vitamin in their diets to avoid mental retardation and epilepsy [1]. More easily diagnosed metabolic problems include disturbed calcium and magnesium handling. Chemical disorders of the blood are routinely sought in the newborn period and usually are easily corrected.

Inbreeding allows some genes to become very common in a closely knit population. This accounts for the high incidence of Tay-Sachs disease in some groups of Ashkenazi Jews (Table 9–3). As much as 3 percent of this population carries the gene that will lead to a deficiency in the enzyme hexosaminidase A [1]. This is a recessively inherited disorder, and so both parents must be carrying the gene for the child to be affected. Children with Tay-Sachs disease

Table 9–3.
Recessively Inherited Metabolic Causes of Epilepsy

Phenylketonuria	Infantile Gaucher disease
Pyridoxine dependency	Metachromatic leukodystrophy
Leigh disease	Krabbe disease
Tay-Sachs disease	Neuronal ceroid lipofuscinosis
Niemann-Pick disease	

develop seizures, retinal damage, and severe mental retardation. This is a lethal disease, in which a victim's survival past 3 years of age is very uncommon. The disorder can be detected early in fetal development, and the parents can be offered the option of terminating the pregnancy before the defective fetus matures [1].

Less common, but equally lethal, metabolic disorders include several defects in lipid or glycogen metabolism. In Niemann-Pick, infantile Gaucher, and Krabbe diseases, material accumulates in nerve cells and causes nervous system damage. In some diseases, this material has a waxy appearance on routine tissue stains, and the disorders are called *neuronal ceroid lipofuscinoses*. All of these unusual metabolic disorders are recessively inherited. There are also several dominantly inherited problems that are fairly common and not invariably lethal [1]. One such metabolic problem is acute intermittent porphyria, an enzyme disorder that may cause intermittent problems with brain function [1].

Most of the X-linked diseases causing seizures are progressive and involve the entire nervous system. Other neurologic signs usually overshadow the seizure disorders, and the victims of these disorders usually die during childhood (Table 9-4) [1]. Treatment of the epilepsy in these patients is frustrating, because the progressive character of the diseases interferes with the development of an effective drug regimen.

Tuberous Sclerosis
Tuberous sclerosis is a hereditary disease that may cause little more than abnormally pigmented spots on the skin or it may induce profound mental retardation and cause epilepsy. This is dominantly inherited, but the extent to which the gene is expressed is variable. One child of every 30,000 to

Table 9–4.
X-Linked Causes of Epilepsy

Menkes steely-hair syndrome
Lesch-Nyhan disease
Adrenoleukodystrophy
Pelizaeus-Merzbacher disease
Hereditary corpus callosum agenesis

100,000 will develop some form of the disease [1]. Common signs with tuberous sclerosis, other than seizures and mental retardation, include whitish spots on the skin, fibromas at the bases of the nails, and tumors in several different organs, including the brain, eye, kidney, and heart [1].

Epilepsy is very common in this disease. Eighty-eight percent of patients with tuberous sclerosis have seizures; this increases to 100 percent if the patient is mentally retarded [1]. Sixty percent of affected individuals are retarded. If seizures appear before the child is 2 years old, that child will be retarded.

Neurofibromatosis
Neurofibromatosis (von Recklinghausen disease) is a hereditary disorder affecting the nervous system as well as the skeleton and skin. It is transmitted in an autosomal dominant pattern and appears in 1 of 3,000 births [1]. Twelve percent of the patients with this disease have seizures, most of which are caused by potentially lethal brain tumors [1]. Individuals with the disorder exhibit lumps in the skin, caused by neurofibromas along nerves in the skin, and hyperpigmented spots called *café au lait spots* that may extend over several centimeters wherever they occur. Dementia does not develop with this disease unless a specific brain lesion, such as a tumor, develops. This condition also has variable penetrance.

Huntington Disease
Although Huntington disease usually causes abnormal movements, progressive dementia, and affective disorders, approximately 10 percent of the patients with this dominantly inherited central nervous system disorder have epilepsy [1]. In the rigid form of this disease, which usually occurs in children or adolescents, there is a much higher incidence of seizure disorders. These children have rigidity, tremor, and bradykinesia similar to the elderly person with Parkinson disease. Approximately 85 percent of children with this rigid form of Huntington disease have epilepsy.

GENETIC COUNSELING

The consequences of genetic counseling have been disturbingly ironic. People informed of the risks of having a child with a hereditary disorder often have more children than people at risk who receive no counseling. The obvious explanation for this phenomenon is that parents of one affected child who are told nothing about risks routinely suspect that any future child will be similarly affected. If they seek help and are told that the chance of having another similarly affected child is only 1 of 4 or 1 of 2, they are more likely to have other children. The attitude seems to be that, even if a second abnormal child is born, the probability of having a normal child is high if they simply continue trying.

Biochemical assays using fetal cells and amniotic fluid have been more helpful than counseling. In many cases, families at risk can be told whether the developing fetus will be affected. Based on this information, the parents can decide whether to continue the pregnancy.

REFERENCES

1. Jennings, M.T., Bird, T.D.   Genetic influences in the epilepsies. *Am. J. Dis. Child.* 135:450–457, 1981.
2. Rosenberg, R.N.   Biochemical genetics of neurologic disease. *N. Engl. J. Med.* 305(20):1181–1193, 1981.
3. Janz, D., Beck-Mannagetta, G., Scheffner, D., et al.   Epilepsy in children of epileptic parents. In Janz, D., Dam, M., Richens, A., et al. (eds.), *Epilepsy, Pregnancy, and the Child.* New York: Raven Press, 1982, pp. 527–534.
4. Tsuboi, T.   Incidence of seizures among offspring of epileptic patients. In Janz, D., Dam, M., Richens, A., et al. (eds.), *Epilepsy, Pregnancy, and the Child.* New York: Raven Press, 1982, pp. 503–507.
5. Blumer, D.   Temporal lobe epilepsy and its psychiatric significance. In Benson, D.F., Blumer, D., Mer, D. (eds.), *Psychiatric Aspects of Neurologic Disease.* New York: Grune & Stratton, 1975, p. 171.
6. Rapin, I.   *Children with Brain Dysfunction. Neurology, Cognition, Language, and Behavior.* New York: Raven Press, 1982, pp. 284.
7. Delgado-Escueta, A.V., Treiman, D.M., Walsh, G.O.   The treatable epilepsies (part 1). *N. Engl. J. Med.* 308(25):1508–1514, 1983.
8. Asconape, J., Penry, J.K.   Some clinical and EEG aspects of benign juvenile myoclonic epilepsy. *Epilepsia* 25(1):108–114, 1984.

10. Children with Epilepsy

Some type of seizure activity occurs in as many as 8 of every 1,000 children [1]. Occasionally, the seizures remit as the child matures, but in most cases, epilepsy appearing in childhood persists into adult life. Approximately 80 percent of all people who have epilepsy at some time in their lives develop the problem while they are children [2]. With well-controlled seizures, the child and his family may face few real problems initiated by the epilepsy; poorly controlled seizures, on the other hand, may exhaust a family's energy and resources [3, 4].

With frequently occurring seizures, parents often feel obliged to restrict the child's life and often their own lives as well [3]. The child himself may be preoccupied with fears that the seizures will cripple or kill him. Even when the seizures are fully controlled, restrictive family interactions that develop as a response to the child's epilepsy may persist long after they are appropriate [5]. A parent's excessive protectiveness may work to the child's advantage when close supervision is essential for seizure control, but that same protectiveness may persist after the seizures stop and, in some families, after the child becomes an adult [5, 6].

LEARNING AND BEHAVIORAL DISORDERS

Children with epilepsy have more behavioral problems and learning disorders than either healthy children or children with other chronic nonneurologic problems, such as respiratory and cardiac diseases [2, 7, 8]. That epilepsy intermittently disturbs brain activity certainly plays a role in the behavioral and learning abnormalities seen in these children, but parental expectations correlate with the child's social and academic performance [8]. Many parents believe their epileptic children are intellectually impaired. Expecting the child to fail to perform at a level appropriate for his age and intelligence helps to ensure that he will fail.

Behavioral problems occur in many different kinds of epilepsy, but children with complex partial and generalized convulsive epilepsy have more difficulty controlling violent or destructive behavior than do children with more focal seizure disorders [7]. Behavioral problems are especially likely in children with complex partial seizures that appear very early in life, particularly if the affected child is male [7, 9]. Although any mention of a behavioral disorder immediately suggests destructive or violent actions, the disorders found in children with complex partial seizures are not invariably aggressive or destructive. Difficulties in socializing with other children, dealing with failure, participating in family activities, and other common demands of childhood appear in these epileptic children.

Violent or destructive behavior does occur in some of these children. Although the most severe behavioral disorders would be expected in individuals burdened with epilepsy from infancy or early childhood, children actually exhibit more violent behavior if they have generalized seizures that first develop relatively late in maturation [9]. Destructive behavior is also common in children with some uncommon types of minor motor seizures, such as akinetic seizures [9]. The reason for this is unknown, just as it is not known why violent behavior in individuals with generalized myoclonic seizures is rare [9].

Psychological, personality, and behavioral disorders of several types are by no means uncommon in children with seizures. When all forms of epilepsy are considered, 25 percent of epileptic children develop psychosocial problems severe enough to justify or require professional attention [2]. These change as the child matures and the overall pattern of change is toward a more self-controlled individual. Psychiatric intervention may be needed over the course of several years [10].

Intellectual Abilities

Learning problems occur at a higher than expected frequency among children with epilepsy. This is not to say that epilepsy and mental retardation are related, a common misconception fostered by the appearance of epilepsy in children with severe mental retardation [2]. The severity of the learning disability these children exhibit is related, at least in part, to the age at which they first have seizures [11]. This may be because disorders that cause both diffuse brain damage and epilepsy are more likely to appear at certain ages (e.g., 0 to 1 year).

Whatever the reason, children 9 to 15 years old with generalized convulsive seizures exhibit less impairment on neuropsychological testing if their seizures first began when they were between 8 and 14 years old rather than before the age of 5 [11]. Tasks requiring simple motor acts, protracted attention, complex problem solving, or good memory function reveal the greatest discrepancy between performances by the children with very early-onset (0 to 5 years of age) and relatively late-onset (after 14 years of age) epilepsies [11].

As a group, the children whose seizures begin before they are 5 years old probably perform more poorly because among them are children who suffered perinatal hypoxia, intrauterine infections, cerebral malformations, and other causes of congenital brain damage. Such brain-damaged children usually have their first seizures before they are 1 year old. The poorer performance evident in children whose first seizures occur before age 5 does not necessarily indicate an adverse effect on the brain of either the seizures themselves or the antiepileptic drugs used to suppress the seizures.

Classroom Problems

Regardless of their intellectual abilities, epileptic children are routinely treated differently from the other children in school. Much of this special treatment is a result of the ways that teachers perceive the children. Even the most understanding teachers are burdened by their own fears and misconceptions about epilepsy. The teacher often worries about inadvertently causing a seizure, and this fear frequently is reinforced by the parents of affected children [2, 4].

Many parents relay grossly inaccurate views of the seizure disorder to the teachers responsible for their children [2]. A mother who has seen her child turn blue during a generalized convulsion may confide in the teacher that the last seizure nearly killed the child. With this type of information, all but the most enlightened teachers will be terrified by the prospect of a seizure occurring in the classroom. Less is demanded of the epileptic children than of their classmates, and the special treatment they are accorded isolates them from the other children.

Epileptic children are commonly described by their teachers as solitary, irritable, uninterested, and unpopular [4]. These children often lag months or years behind their peers academically as well as socially, and most teachers ascribe this slow advancement to medication effects, parental attitudes, and even their own attitudes toward the children [4]. Children with epilepsy do less well in school than would be expected from psychological and intelligence tests [8]. At least part of this underachievement results from parental attitudes and behavior [8].

Parental Attitudes

Parents often infantilize children with epilepsy even after adolescence [12]. They expect their children to perform less well than schoolchildren without epilepsy in social activities, sports, and future employment, and they emphasize the disabilities ascribed to their epileptic children by having the children excused from sports and other strenuous activities [8]. This not only announces the child's problem to his peers, but also reinforces the social isolation that is characteristically accepted by the affected child [2, 8].

Many parents admit that they see their epileptic child as an unfortunate person who cannot and should not be expected to achieve anything [2]. The child with epilepsy often incorporates his parents' view of most things, including their view of him [2, 12]. Expectations are inappropriately limited, and these children generally behave dependently in interpersonal relationships [12].

Hyperactivity

When children are excessively active, easily distracted, unable to concentrate on anything for more than a few minutes, and insensitive to all efforts to moderate their activity level, they are called *hyperactive* [13]. This behavior sometimes develops in children with epilepsy, and in many cases, it is an adverse reaction to antiepileptic medication (see Chapter 14). Regardless of its cause, hyperactivity may interfere substantially with the child's education.

If the antiepileptic medication is responsible for the hyperactivity, other drugs must be tried to find which produces the least disturbing behavior. Of course, there are some children with epilepsy in whom the hyperactivity is unrelated to medication or seizure activity. In children in whom there is no apparent structural lesion, the temper tantrums, hyperactivity, and poor frustration tolerance generally improve with age [14]. Children with persistent or increasing hyperactivity who do not respond to medication changes or maturation usually have structural damage to the brain. Structural brain damage and intellectual impairment secondary to undocumented brain damage are more closely tied to hyperactivity and destructiveness in children than is any social factor [14].

FAMILY PROBLEMS

Epilepsy in a child unavoidably disturbs relationships in the family [15]. This starts with the child's self-image and extends to the way every member of the family sees the child. Rather than developing a sense of control over the inanimate world—that is, a sense of competence—early in life, the epileptic child experiences a less than normal level of control over the forces acting on him [3]. Parents, too, are unable to exert much control over the epilepsy that intimately affects daily activity. This is especially important, because in any family, fear and security are routinely magnified in the exchange between the child and his parents [3, 8, 16, 17]. Those things feared by his parents seem even more ominous to the child than the things that the child intuitively finds frightening. As a reaction to fear and impotence, the parents may worry about the child's health, strenuously deny the child's problem, or simply reject the chronically impaired individual.

The parents' behavior toward the epileptic child commonly involves an element of shame [8]. This embarrassment over having an impaired child rarely is overt, but it usually is apparent enough to be felt by the child [8]. At least in part because of this parental shame, the child often exhibits a reluctance to venture outside the family and has a poor self-image [15].

When parents fail to deal constructively with the child's epilepsy, the failure can often be traced to their own prejudices about this neurologic disorder [2]. Regardless of education or socioeconomic class, the epileptic child's parents are routinely burdened with mystical or archaic ideas about the causes of epilepsy [2]. Often, they believe that the seizures were imposed on their child by malevolent forces or a demanding god, and they react to the seizure disorder in an indulgent or demanding manner [8].

Any approach to managing the child must change as the child ages or the seizures change in character. The degree to which the parents are inflexible in approaching the epilepsy directly affects the extent of the problem caused by the epilepsy at a very practical level. This is obvious in the rate of seizure control seen in different types of families. Children with autocratic parents have a poorer response to therapeutic doses of antiepileptic drugs than do children with less restrictive parents [8]. Children generally have fewer problems with seizure control if they are from families that allow the child to develop with a reasonable level of independence and discipline.

Parents are usually unfamiliar with what is happening to their child but rarely seek authoritative information on the subject [8]. One-third of parents with epileptic children never frankly discuss the child's seizures with him or her. The parents are frightened by the seizures and routinely admit that they have no idea of what to do when a seizure occurs, even if they have had the opportunity to discuss the disorder with a physician [8]. More than half never read anything about the epilepsy, but they do gather considerable hearsay from friends and relatives [8]. Consequently, they treat their epileptic children the way they would any sick child [2], although clearly, what is appropriate for an illness lasting days or weeks is not applicable for a disorder that lasts years or a lifetime.

Children quickly realize that parental fears and guilt are easily played upon [3]. Efforts to discipline the children can be subverted by the fear that such treatment will cause a seizure [2]. This intimidation of the parents aggravates an already difficult family situation and produces considerable resentment, a resentment that usually is not recognized by the individuals involved. The struggle to control the child becomes more oppressive, under the guise of protecting the patient. Excitement may be banned because of the risk of seizures [2, 16]. All opportunities to fail, even if that failure will be instructive, are eliminated.

The child with frequent seizures imposes restrictions on the family that may make the child a virtual tyrant. All of the family's activities may be tailored to the child's limitations. Many parents become angry over the restrictions imposed by their child, but, in dealing with the child, they may react more to the guilt they feel because of this anger than to the anger itself [3]. They fail to develop enough confidence, in the face of the neurologic disorder, to tell the child what to do. Rather than becoming adversaries of the epileptic child, the parents may acquiesce to the patient's every whim, always adopting the position that they only want to do what is best for him or her [3].

The child who appreciates the power he exerts over his family because of the epilepsy soon realizes that the seizures do not have to be unpredictable or even real to be effective. Children quickly learn what will provoke a seizure and may use that to their advantage [2]. Children can also have factitious seizures when a self-induced attack is impossible. This will force the most unbending parent to compromise, but it does have the disadvantage of excluding the child from many activities that he might enjoy.

Parents often react to their inability to control or eliminate the child's epilepsy by intruding extraordinarily into the affected child's life [3]. As many as 1 of 3 parents of epileptic children believe that their children require constant supervision, even after the seizures have been completely controlled for months or years [8]. Parents encourage passivity and discourage initiative in these offspring [8]. Eating habits, friendships, travel patterns, and play may be harshly regulated. There is legitimate concern that the seizures will occur in a dangerous situation, and so the child's opportunity to explore is severely restricted [6].

Families with epileptic children function as more disciplined units than families without similarly affected children. This is true even after the child has been seizure-free for more than 6 months [5]. Problems are solved in an efficient, albeit tyrannical, manner. The hierarchy in these families is much more evident and rigid than in families without epileptic children. In it, the child's mother assumes an inordinately dominant position if she is primarily responsible for the child [5]. Apparently, this rigid family structure not only serves the child's needs to be protected and supervised, but it also minimizes the disruptive influence of the epilepsy [5]. Eventually the child either rebels to all controls exerted on him or he becomes devastatingly passive and dependent on the restrictive parents [3, 6]. These responses to restrictions usually are misinterpreted by the parents as facets of the epilepsy or reactions to the medication, and the responsible physician is expected to manage the problem [6].

Dealing with children with poorly controlled epilepsy is not simple, but there are some techniques that minimize the difficulties encountered. The physician should try to make all members of the immediate family aware of precisely what the child's problem is. Fantasies must be explored and rejected if they are inaccurate [3]. Attempts to place blame on one member of the family or another must be discouraged. Accusations of this sort are poorly disguised attempts to reject any responsibility for the epilepsy.

The child's abilities should be objectively assessed and exploited. As the child matures, he should be allowed and encouraged to be responsible for monitoring his own activities and taking his own medication. The child should deal directly with the primary physician as soon as this is practical. The ways in which the family behaves toward the patient must change as the patient changes. If parents and siblings cannot make the changes needed to interact productively with the patient, they may profit from family therapy [15].

PROBLEMS WITH ADOLESCENT COMPLIANCE

The principal concerns of most children during adolescence are independence, identity, and conformity, and all of these are complicated by the epilepsy and its treatment [2]. In many Western countries, part of the independence that comes with adolescence is the autonomy provided by driving a car or motorcycle. If epilepsy is still an active problem, it will necessarily curtail the individual's ability to drive.

Some adolescents solve this problem by simply denying that they have epilepsy. Not having epilepsy means not taking medication, a practice that is usually identified with overbearing parents anyway. The epileptic adolescent often tries to be independent by abandoning the precautions enforced by his parents [3]. This makes good seizure control very difficult.

Another common problem that develops during adolescence is drug abuse. In a culture prone to drug abuse, the unlimited access to controlled drugs provides an easy route to popularity. Ironically, the same adolescent that resists family pressure to take the antiepileptic medications may experiment with excessive doses of the drugs. Changing to antiepileptics with no resale value or well-recognized abuse potential minimizes this behavior.

Although alcohol and other types of drug abuse are not limited to adolescence, they are likely to start at that age. These substances alter the metabolism of antiepileptic drugs, and so extra care must be taken to ensure that the serum medication level stays within the therapeutic range. If the substance abuse has been well concealed by the patient, the parents may present the child to the physician with extreme anxiety over the abrupt resurgence of epileptic activity. Whenever seizure control deteriorates during adolescence, the physician will find that dealing directly with the child is more informative and profitable than trying to manage the case through the parents.

PROGNOSIS

Even before anticonvulsants were used, many seizure disorders remitted within months or years of their appearance [14]. Currently, as many as 85 percent of patients who consult a physician within a year of the appearance of a possible seizure do not develop a chronic seizure disorder [14]. This drops to 50 percent for patients who do not consult a physician until seizures have recurred several times over the course of at least 1 year. Although these figures represent many people who have isolated seizures unrelated to epilepsy, they do suggest that if the seizures are going to remit, they will usually do so within a year of their appearance [14].

Different types of epilepsy exhibit different rates of remission. Generalized absence seizures often abate late in adolescence and leave the patient free of focal neurologic deficits and dementia [14]. Infantile spasms, on the other hand, may abate, but they often are replaced by other seizure types and are routinely associated with devastating neurologic deficits in the children who survive after these infantile spasms abate [14]. Antiepileptic medications have not substantially affected the remission rates of different types of epilepsy [14].

Risk of Recurrence after One Seizure

Some seizures are not very likely to recur, and so there is controversy over whether they should be treated. The simple febrile seizure is an example of this, and the current consensus is that children who experience only one or two of these seizures should not be given antiepileptic medication. Complicating the decision on when and whether to treat some types of seizures is the problem of identifying seizures in infants and young children. These patients cannot be relied on to provide histories, and so there are children who have many seizures before epilepsy is suspected. The initial absence attack or myoclonic seizure usually goes unnoticed or is ascribed to fatigue or restlessness. These seizures should be treated when they are recognized.

More controversial is what should be done for a child who has his first generalized tonic-clonic, focal sensory, focal motor, or complex partial seizure. The approximate risk of subsequent seizures can be estimated according to the cause of the seizure, the incidence of epilepsy in the family, and the electroencephalographic pattern observed after the child has recovered from the seizure [18]. The age at which the child develops his first seizure, the type of seizure observed, and the neurologic abnormalities evident at the time of the first seizure are not particularly helpful in determining whether more seizures will occur [18]. Even if the first seizure episode is status epilepticus, subsequent seizure activity need not develop.

If there is no apparent cause for the seizures, even in the presence of focal neurologic abnormalities on the patient's examination, the likelihood that another seizure will occur within 3 years of the first seizure is 26 percent [18]. If the patient had a neurologic injury, such as meningitis or head trauma, the risk of recurrence within 3 years is 34 percent [18]. Patients whose brothers or sisters have epilepsy have a seizure recurrence rate of 35 percent within

4 months of the initial attack [18]. If the seizure develops after massive head trauma, the risk of a second seizure is 46 percent by 20 months. Seizures that are caused by nervous system problems other than head trauma will recur within 20 months in 28 percent of cases [18]. With any of these risk factors, antiepileptic drug treatment is favored over just observing the child.

Predictors of Seizure Recurrence
Although the electroencephalogram is not particularly useful in predicting which patients will remain seizure-free after several years without seizures, it is helpful in identifying patients likely to have epilepsy after one seizure episode. A generalized spike–and–slow wave pattern on the electroencephalogram hours or days after the patient has recovered from the seizure is correlated with a high probability of more seizure activity within days or months. Individuals with this electroencephalographic abnormality will have another seizure within 18 months of the first seizure in approximately 50 percent of cases [18]. With spikes over the central temporal area, the risk of recurrent seizures is even greater [18]. Unsuspected lesions may be revealed by a slow wave focus (Fig. 10–1) on a routine electroencephalogram. If the patient has evidence of structural brain disease, antiepileptic medication should be given while the nature of the lesion is investigated. If the electroencephalogram is normal or has nonspecific abnormalities after an idiopathic seizure, the likelihood that a second seizure will occur within 2 years is 14 percent.

Effect of Therapy
The risk of recurrence is not substantially affected by the prescription of antiepileptic medications, but this may be because patients do not usually take this medication faithfully after only one seizure has occurred [18]. In fact, most physicians would not prescribe antiepileptic drugs after only one seizure, because of the distinct possibility that another seizure will never occur whether or not the patient is treated. Once the medication is started, the patient is committed to years of treatment, unless it can subsequently be proved that the seizure was symptomatic of a transient disorder, such as hypocalcemia, that is not expected to recur unpredictably.

Long-term Treatment

Some types of childhood seizure disorders are clearly self-limited. For instance, by the end of adolescence, the child with rolandic seizures will be seizure-free [4]. However, most seizure disorders are not that predictable. Deciding when or whether to stop antiepileptic drugs is no simple matter in these less predictable epilepsies.

The child's condition while still on medication is the single most important consideration in deciding how long the drugs should be continued. If the child has poorly controlled seizures while taking antiepileptic drugs or requires a

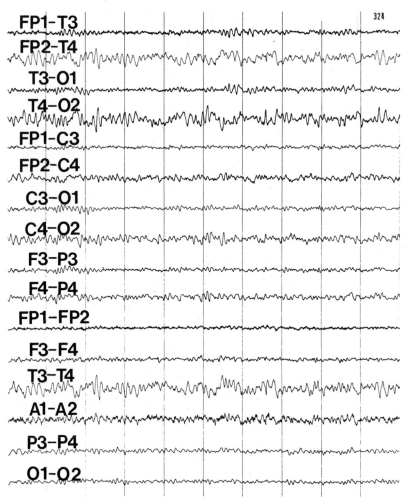

Figure 10–1.

This electroencephalogram revealed a structural lesion in the temporofrontal region, demonstrated by slow waves (a delta focus) evident in the electrode pairs that include T4. (FP = frontoparietal; T = temporal; O = occipital; C = central; F = frontal; P = parietal; A = ear.)

combination of medications to suppress the seizures, it is not appropriate to stop the drug use. After seizures have been suppressed for more than 3 or 4 years, both the parents and the affected child often are eager to try managing without any further antiepileptic treatment. In any particular case, all that can be offered the patient or his parents is the probability that seizures will not recur if all medication is stopped. If the child has had no seizures for 4 years while using one antiepileptic drug, he will remain seizure-free off all medication in 72 percent of cases [19]. Of the 28 percent with renewed seizure activity after the drugs are stopped, 85 percent have the relapse within the first 5 years after the drugs are stopped, and 56 percent have the relapse during the first year [19]. The risk of relapse is greatest if the child had several years of poor seizure control before the attacks were completely suppressed.

Other factors that make remission of the epilepsy less likely include unequivocal central nervous system damage associated with the seizures and the presence of multiple seizure types in the affected child [19]. With focal motor and jacksonian seizures, the attacks invariably recur when medications are stopped, and so discontinuation of the drugs is inadvisable for the child with these seizure types [19].

Although the reliability of electroencephalographic studies in predicting long-term patterns of epilepsy is controversial, there is evidence that certain electroencephalographic patterns indicate better prognoses than others. In some instances, the brain wave evidence simply reiterates the predictions that can be made from clinical signs alone. Half the children with the electroencephalographic pattern characteristic of rolandic seizures will have no seizures or electrical abnormalities on repeated tests by the time they are 15 years old [14]. Deciding that the child actually has benign focal epilepsy of childhood (rolandic epilepsy) is greatly influenced by the patient's clinical signs, and so the electroencephalogram is not very informative.

With an occipital lobe focus on the electroencephalogram, 48 percent of children will be seizure-free by the time they are 9 years old [14]. This does not mean that the child will never have another seizure. Long-term follow-up of patients who are off medication and who have no seizures usually is limited to only a few years.

Although an abnormal electroencephalogram may be helpful in establishing the risk of recurrent seizures shortly after the child has his first seizure, it is not helpful in predicting relapses after drugs are stopped [19]. Seizure relapse is no more common in children with persistently abnormal electroencephalograms than in those with normal records. The number of seizures the patient had before control was achieved also does not indicate the probability that he will remain seizure-free off all medication. The child's age when the seizures first appeared, his age when the medication is stopped, the sex of the child, and a family history of epilepsy are also not helpful in predicting the likelihood that he will remain seizure-free [19]. The ways in which the seizures evolved and the type of epilepsy the child eventuallly exhibited do help predict the risk of recurrent seizures if drug treatment is discontinued. Children who have had a febrile seizure followed by a nonfebrile seizure usually need drugs to stay seizure-free, even after no seizures have occurred for more than 4 years. Patients with the best chance of remaining seizure-free off medication after 4 years of complete control are those with idiopathic generalized epilepsies [19].

Onset in Infancy

Seizures that begin at a very early age are no more likely to have a poor prognosis than seizures developing later in childhood, unless those seizures are infantile spasms [20, 21]. This means that the child who has a seizure at 1 year of age is at no more risk of developing epilepsy or mental retardation than the child whose first seizure occurs at 7 years of age [20]. The child's prognosis is affected by neurologic problems that were evident before the seizures occurred.

There are particular seizure types that usually occur in infancy and are associated with a poor prognosis, but the determining factor in these cases is the pattern of epilepsy, not the age of the child. Infants with infantile spasms or other types of minor motor seizures often develop mental retardation, but even in these children, neurologic deficits usually are apparent in the affected children even before the seizures occur [20]. Half of the children with seizures in whom mental retardation is evident by the time they are 7 years old are found to have had minor motor seizures, infantile spasms, or obvious neurologic deficits in infancy [20]. Twenty-seven percent of the children who have nonfebrile seizures by the time they are 7 years old have an intelligence quotient (I.Q.) lower than 70 [20]. Children with neurologic problems are simply more likely to develop seizures than children unburdened by these central nervous system disorders.

Seizures do not necessarily develop as an early sign of brain damage, but they may. Children with neurologic abnormalities evident by 1 year of age develop seizures no sooner than children without apparent neurologic deficits [20]. However, that an infant has evidence of brain damage greatly increases the probability that the patient will have seizures at some time during childhood. Twenty-one percent of children with febrile seizures and 40 percent with nonfebrile seizures have neurologic problems, such as weakness, delayed psychomotor development, or sensory deficits, by the time they are 1 year old [20].

Neonatal Seizures
Approximately 15 percent of the infants who have neonatal seizures die during infancy or early childhood [22]. Of those who survive, 35 percent have mental retardation, motor deficits, or epilepsy [22]. As with any type of epilepsy, the cause of the central nervous system disorder plays a major role in determining the prognosis, and many of the causes of neonatal seizures are lethal. Infants with neonatal seizures following hypoxic or ischemic damage to the brain have only a 10 to 20 percent chance for apparently normal development [22]. Those who develop seizures after an unexplained subarachnoid hemorrhage—that is, one not caused by bleeding from an arteriovenous malformation or tumor—have a 90 percent chance of developing normally [22].

Brain wave patterns in these very small children have more prognostic value than those observed later in childhood. If the interictal electroencephalogram is normal in the full-term infant with neonatal seizures, the child usually does well in terms of survival and psychomotor development. Eighty-six percent of the children with grossly normal interictal brain waves develop normally at least until they are 4 years old, and probably after that. Those whose electroencephalograms reveal multifocal abnormalities develop normally in only 12 percent of cases [22]. Certain electroencephalographic patterns, such as burst suppression, are associated with especially poor prognoses. None of these brain wave findings are helpful in predicting the outcome if the infant is premature.

Controlling neonatal seizures probably does affect the outcome for the child. There is evidence that frequent seizures in the neonate can cause brain damage or disturbed brain development [22]. It remains to be determined which anticonvulsant is least likely to interfere with brain maturation and provide the most protection from recurrent seizures (see Chapter 14).

Infantile Spasms
Infantile spasms usually appear after the neonatal period, but they, too, have a very poor prognosis. As discussed in Chapter 14, the outlook is better if children with infantile spasms are treated within the first month of spasms with high-dose adrenocorticotropic hormone [21]. Regardless of the treatment used, these children often die or survive with severe mental retardation and epilepsy [21]. If the child has spasms because of tuberous sclerosis, meningoencephalitis, intrauterine asphyxia, or another readily definable destructive lesion in the brain, the prognosis will reflect the severity of the underlying disease. Even if the infantile spasms are idiopathic, the likelihood that the child will develop normally and have no seizures at a later date is less than 15 percent (Table 10–1). Most infants will show developmental delays within weeks of the first infantile spasm if they do not already exhibit such delays by the time the infantile spasms start [21].

Fewer than 10 percent of children with infantile spasms develop the problem after they are 11 months old, and the worst prognosis is seen in those children who develop the seizures before 3 months of age [21]. Other factors associated with a high probability of retardation and epilepsy are female sex and neonatal seizures. If the infant had another type of seizure before the spasms appeared or the child develops another pattern of epilepsy while the spasms are still

Table 10–1.
Factors Suggesting Poor Prognosis With Infantile Spasms

Onset of spasms before 3 months of age
Appearance of psychomotor delays before infantile spasms begin
History of neonatal seizures
Concurrent development of other seizure types
Atypical electroencephalogram
Female sex

---

evident, the prognosis is extremely poor [21]. Most children cry after a cluster of infantile spasms, but some make a laughing noise or appear to smile; those without the typical crying do more poorly [21].

The electroencephalographic pattern usually seen with infantile spasms is hypsarrhythmia, a diffusely disorganized high-voltage record, but some infants exhibit other types of abnormalities even though their episodes are indistinguishable from typical infantile spasms. The children with atypical electroencephalograms do worse than those with hypsarrhythmia [21]. The electroencephalographic pattern invariably changes as the child matures, but the pattern of change has no prognostic value [21].

More than 50 percent of the children who survive with infantile spasms will continue to have seizures [21]. In most cases, these are generalized tonic-clonic seizures, but some are tonic, atonic, or focal. Twenty to 25 percent of infants with infantile spasms subsequently develop Lennox-Gastaut syndrome (see Chapter 2). The type of treatment used does not affect the type of epilepsy that develops. With the early administration of adrenocorticotropic hormone, seizures are slightly less likely to develop after the infantile spasms abate. Infantile spasms usually stop by the time the child is 3 years old.

Generalized Absence Epilepsy

The natural history of generalized absence epilepsy is better understood than that of most other childhood seizure disorders, simply because it is common and fairly easily identified. Seizures often remit with this type of epilepsy, and even when spontaneous remission does not occur, the probability that the child will have good seizure control on routine antiepileptic drugs is fairly predictable.

Children with generalized absence seizures followed for 10 years are free of all types of epilepsy in 48 percent of cases; of those who have persistent seizures 58 percent are free of their absence seizures but have other types of epilepsy, such as benign juvenile myoclonic, complex partial, or generalized tonic-clonic [23]. At least three-fourths of the patients in whom seizures no longer occur require no medication to remain seizure-free, and so they are accurately considered to have had remissions [23]. Absence seizures are classified into several different subtypes depending on whether the child loses muscle tone, has increased tone, or exhibits subtle automatisms during the seizures (see Table 1–2), but the subtype does not affect the likelihood of remission [23].

If the child has strictly absence attacks, without associated tonic-clonic or myoclonic seizures, the likelihood that seizures will remit within 10 years is 64 percent; if other seizure types appear along with the absence seizures, this probability of remission falls to 34 percent [23]. Several patient characteristics invariably improve the prognosis with this type of epilepsy. If the child has an I.Q. of greater than 90 or has a normal neurologic examination on several

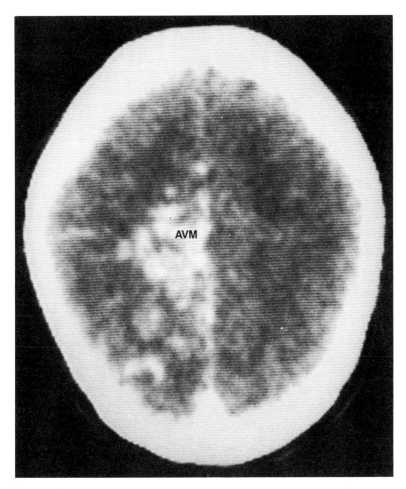

Figure 10–2.
This child had epilepsy because of an unresectable arteriovenous malformation (AVM).
Although her generalized tonic-clonic seizures were infrequent, her underlying brain
disease severely limited her life expectancy.

occasions separated by years, the outlook for complete remission of the epilepsy without the appearance of another type of epilepsy is good. The prognosis is also better for patients whose other family members have no seizure disorders [23]. Considering diagnostic and clinical features of the patient and his epilepsy, one can predict a better than 90 percent chance that the seizure will remit if the child has a normal I.Q., is a boy, has a normal neurologic examination, and exhibits no spike-and-wave complexes on the electroencephalogram with hyperventilation [23].

The electroencephalographic pattern alone does not have prognostic value in this type of epilepsy, but as one of several variables, it assumes significance. Looking at the patterns of seizures exhibited by the patient, one finds that in patients who never exhibit generalized tonic-clonic seizures, the prognosis for normal development and remission of seizures is better than in children who have these seizures mixed with absence attacks [23].

Factors that play no role in the prognosis with generalized absence seizures include the age of the mother at conception, the duration of gestation, and the birth weight of the infant [23]. Absence seizures are not the result of a perinatal injury. The age at which the child first develops the absence attacks also does not affect the prognosis [23]. If the child develops absence status epilepticus at any time, the outlook for remission of the seizures is poor, but this type of status epilepticus is rare [23].

That seizures remit for months or even years does not guarantee that the child with absence seizures will never have seizures again. In fact, 11 to 12 percent of patients who become seizure-free after a history of childhood absence attacks will experience a relapse of seizure activity after a protracted seizure-free interval [23].

Mortality

The risk of early death in children with idiopathic epilepsy is fairly small. Increased mortality is associated with symptomatic epilepsies in which a progressive or lethal nervous system disorder is responsible for the epilepsy and other neurologic problems (Fig. 10–2). The higher mortality found among young people with epilepsy without progressive brain disease is attributable to status epilepticus, accidents, and suicide [24, 25]. Suicide attempts are not particularly common in children, although poor drug compliance may lead to inadvertent deaths. Accidents are very common among epileptic children and adolescents, but if the accident is fatal, it often is impossible to determine whether the epilepsy or antiepileptic medication played a role.

REFERENCES

1. Berg, B.O. Prognosis of childhood epilepsy—another look. *N. Engl. J. Med.* 306(14):861–862, 1982.
2. Appolone, C. Preventive social work intervention with families of children with epilepsy. *Soc. Work Health Care* 4(2):139–148, 1978.
3. Ziegler, R.G. Impairments of control and competence in epileptic children and their families. *Epilepsia* 22:339–346, 1981.
4. Burden, G. Social aspects. In Reynolds, E.H., Trimble, M.R. (eds.), *Epilepsy and Psychiatry.* New York: Churchill Livingstone, 1981, pp. 296–305.
5. Ritchie, K. Research note: interaction in the families of epileptic children. *J. Child Psychol. Psychiatry* 22:65–71, 1981.

6. Pond, D. Psycho-social aspects of epilepsy—the family. In Reynolds, E.H., Trimble, M.R., *Epilepsy and Psychiatry.* New York: Churchill Livingstone, 1981, pp. 291–295.
7. Hermann, B.P., Black, R.B., Chhabria, S. Behavioral problems and social competence in children with epilepsy. *Epilepsia* 22:703–710, 1981.
8. Long, C.G., Moore, J.R. Parental expectations for their epileptic children. *J. Child Psychol. Psychiatry* 20:299–312, 1979.
9. Hermann, B.P., Schwartz, M.S., Whitman, S., et al. Aggression and epilepsy: seizure-type comparisons and high-risk variables. *Epilepsia* 21:691–698, 1980.
10. Lechtenberg, R. *The Psychiatrist's Guide to Diseases of the Nervous System.* New York: John Wiley & Sons, 1982.
11. O'Leary, D.S., Seidenberg, M., Berent, S., et al. Effects of age of onset of tonic-clonic seizures on neuropsychological performance in children. *Epilepsia* 22:197–204, 1981.
12. Lessman, S.E., Mollick, L.R. Group treatment of epileptics. *Health Soc. Work* 3(3):106–121, 1978.
13. Denckla, M.B., Heilman, K.M. The syndrome of hyperactivity. In Heilman, K.M., Valenstein, E. (eds.), *Clinical Neuropsychology.* New York: Oxford University Press, 1979, p. 574.
14. Rodin, E.A. *The Prognosis of Patients with Epilepsy.* Springfield, Ill.: Charles C Thomas, 1968, p. 455.
15. Lechtenberg, R. *Epilepsy and The Family.* Cambridge, Mass.: Harvard University Press, 1984.
16. Berney, T.P., Osselto, J.W., Kelvin, I., et al. Effects of discotheque environment on epileptic children. *Br. Med. J.* 282(6259):180–182, 1981.
17. Lamb, M.E. Paternal influences on early socio-emotional development. *J. Child Psychol. Psychiatry* 23:185–190, 1982.
18. Hauser, W.A., Anderson, V.E., Loewenson, R.B., et al. Seizure recurrence after a first unprovoked seizure. *N. Engl. J. Med.* 307(9):522–528, 1982.
19. Thurston, J.H., Thurston, D.L., Hixon, B.B., et al. Prognosis in childhood epilepsy. *N. Engl. J. Med.* 306(14):831–836, 1982.
20. Ellenberg, J.H., Hirtz, D.G., Nelson, K.B. Age at onset of seizures in young children. *Ann. Neurol.* 15(2):127–134, 1984.
21. Lombroso, C.T. A prospective study of infantile spasms: clinical and therapeutic correlations. *Epilepsia* 24(2):135–158, 1983.
22. Volpe, J.J. Neonatal seizures. *Clin. Perinatol.* 4(1):43–63, 1977.
23. Sato, S., Dreifuss, F.E., Penry, J.K., et al. Long-term follow-up of absence seizures. *Neurology* (N.Y.) 33:1590–1595, 1983.
24. Hauser, W.A., Annegers, J.F., Elvebac, L.R. Mortality in patients with epilepsy. *Epilepsia* 21:399–412, 1980.
25. Barraclough, B. Suicide and epilepsy. In Reynolds, E.H., Trimble, M.R. (eds.), *Epilepsy and Psychiatry.* New York: Churchill Livingstone, 1981, pp. 72–76.

11. Psychological Disturbances and Suicide

Psychological problems occur with all chronic illnesses, and epilepsy is no exception. Still unresolved after several decades of controversy is the question of which types of psychological problems or changes occur in people with epilepsy. The controversy centers on whether there is anything truly characteristic about the personality, mood, and behavioral patterns occurring with any or all types of epilepsy. Some patients are depressed as a reaction to the problem, and some may even have peculiar notions about the cause of their disorder, but this is true of patients with any chronic condition. As with other chronic medical problems, there is a slight but disturbing increase in the incidence of suicide among epileptic individuals. It has been repeatedly suggested by some neurologists, and refuted by others, that there are distinct patterns of psychopathology and sociopathy associated with some forms of epilepsy and not with others. This has been an especially heated controversy, because many physicians oppose the popular notion that there is something emotionally or intellectually different about people with epilepsy. The suggestion by other physicians that people with complex partial seizures or other types of seizures are prone to violence, sexual perversions, or more subtle affective disorders undermines years of work to change the warped view of epilepsy held by the general public.

From the arguments over the psychological profile of patients with epilepsy we have learned that there are some personality traits and behavioral patterns that occur more often in individuals with certain types of epilepsy than in the general population. In some cases, these psychological characteristics are clearly pathologic; in most cases, they are not. That the epilepsy is responsible for the characteristics has not been established. That any will occur in a particular individual with a specific type of epilepsy is impossible to predict.

The reluctance of physicians to associate any affective or behavioral changes with epilepsy is understandable, since a principal objective in dealing with any patient is to emphasize ways to eliminate problems imposed by the disorder rather than to belabor the types of problems the patient may eventually face. However, if particular types of mood or behavioral disturbances can be associated with the seizures, or even with the level of seizure control, the patient can be spared excessive investigations and the physician can manage more directly and effectively any problems that arise. The epileptic patient will not necessarily experience psychological problems or changes, but those that do arise require specific approaches that take into account the significance of the patient's seizure disorder.

PERSONALITY TRAITS

At least 75 percent of patients with epilepsy have some type of intellectual, affective, behavioral, or simply neurologic problem [1]. This problem may be nothing more than a reactive depression, or it may be severe mental retardation. The fraction of the epileptic population with some problem is so large because it includes all patients with seizures from structural or metabolic brain diseases, who are impaired because of their brain disease and not necessarily because of their epilepsy.

Approximately half of the epileptic population has psychological or social problems that are manifest in daily activities and behavior [1]. Depression, excessive anxiety, self-denigration, hypochondriasis, confused thinking, excessive sensitivity, and pervasive dissatisfaction are commonly reported by and observed in adults with epilepsy. The individual with epilepsy usually exhibits several of these characteristics or none at all. In other words, most patients who are depressed are also anxious and overly sensitive.

If such personality traits appear abruptly, it is important for the primary physician to consider structural, infectious, or metabolic bases for the change. Even people with epilepsy can develop a chronic subdural hematoma, frontal lobe glioma, bacterial meningitis, or diabetes mellitus. These must be sought before any less acute etiologies are considered (Fig. 11–1).

If structural, infectious, or metabolic lesions are not responsible for the psychological problems, social factors may play a large role. Psychosocial profiles show that many people with epilepsy are embarrassed when their seizures occur, resent having this problem, feel that their worth is diminished by it, and believe that they are less accepted by others because of their condition [1]. These feelings are unfortunate, but none of them is pathologic. Even the

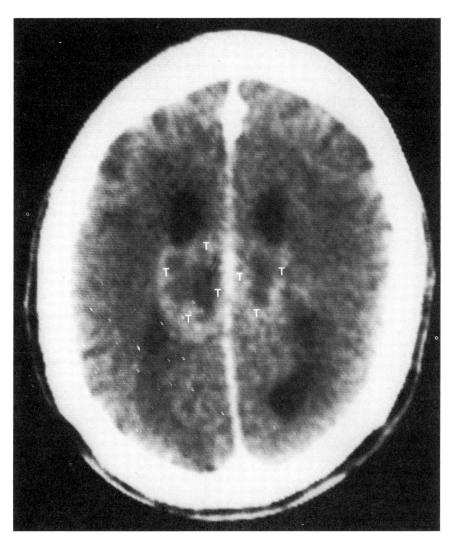

Figure 11–1.
The most obvious neurologic sign exhibited by the man on whom this computed tomogram was obtained was a progressive personality disorder. This proved to be caused by a glioma (T) extending into both frontal lobes from the midline.

patients who experience these emotions are not necessarily deterred by them. Seventy percent of patients with epilepsy see themselves as neither particularly limited nor subject to special treatment because of their seizures [2]. Many are indifferent to the alienation that some people exhibit when they discover the patient has epilepsy, and these patients are the ones most likely to achieve a fairly normal life-style.

Psychopathology in Epilepsy

The type of epilepsy most often implicated in studies of psychopathology with seizure disorders is complex partial epilepsy. The patients specifically identified as exhibiting unusually high rates of psychoses and personality disorders are those with seizures arising in the temporal lobes. Of all patients with epilepsy and an unequivocal history of psychosis, 60 to 70 percent have temporal lobe foci for their seizures [3]. However, this is not an extraordinarily large fraction of the adult epileptic population, since as many as 65 percent of adult patients with epilepsy have complex partial seizures that apparently originate in the temporal lobes. More impressive is the relative paucity of psychopathology in patients with focal motor, focal sensory, and jacksonian seizures [3]. All of these are also partial seizures. That psychological problems are overrepresented in one type suggests that there is something unusual about the effect of that type of epilepsy on the brain or there is something detrimental about the types and locations of lesions that give rise to complex partial seizures.

Personality Disorders in Childhood

Psychological problems and changes occur most commonly in patients with complex partial epilepsy who had their first seizures during adolescence. Developing these seizures before or after results in a lower overall rate of personality disorders [4]. This may be due to the exaggerated impact in adolescence of problems that interfere with the development of a stable self-image, or it may have more to do with the types of cerebral lesions that precipitate seizures at this age.

Children with seizure foci in the temporal lobes exhibit an unusually high incidence of social maladjustment, but this is more clearly correlated with intellectual problems than with seizure activity. Epileptic children with low scores on tests of cognitive function exhibit high levels of aggressive behavior, poor competence in social settings, and a variety of associated behavioral disorders [5]. Unprovoked rage and hyperactivity occur most often in epileptic children with extensive brain damage [5], which suggests that the important factor in personality and behavioral disorders, at least in children, is the brain injury or dysfunction that underlies the epilepsy rather than the epilepsy itself. This is more than an academic distinction: If brain damage produces these personality and behavioral disorders, then seizure control is not likely to affect them.

The lesion responsible for the epilepsy need not be in the temporal lobe and need not be apparent to be associated with obvious behavioral or personality disorders. Children with benign juvenile myoclonic epilepsy, an idiopathic epilepsy in which absence, myoclonic, and tonic-clonic seizures often occur at one time or another, have a higher than expected incidence of behavioral disorders [6]. The character traits that seem to be exaggerated in these adolescents include a lack of self-discipline and a remarkable indifference to limitations, such as those imposed by their neurologic disorder [6]. Whether these character traits persist or change as the patient becomes an adult is uncertain.

Adult Patterns of Psychopathology

The psychopathology that occurs in epileptic adults is seen primarily in individuals with complex partial seizures. Because many of the personality and behavioral disorders occurring in these patients have been labeled *schizophrenic* or *schizophreniform,* the inaccurate impression has developed that this psychopathology is the same or similar to that seen in people with strictly functional psychoses. The functional psychoses may yet prove to be caused by some identifiable brain lesion or disorder, but epilepsy clearly will not be one of those identifiable disorders. Patients with epilepsy and schizophrenia have two very different problems. Patients with the types of psychopathology that develop in a significant proportion of epileptic individuals do not have schizophrenia [7, 8].

Identifying personality disorders, character traits, and persistent mood disturbances that are not simply postictal signs may be difficult in patients with frequent or subtle seizures. Patients with seizures originating in the temporal lobes may have language problems, such as word-finding difficulties, persisting long after what is clearly the postictal period [9]. Much of the peculiar behavior attributed to individuals with seizures originating in the temporal lobes may be from an unbalanced recovery of neurologic functions during the hours or days following a seizure.

Characterizing the population with epilepsy, or even that with complex partial epilepsy, as more susceptible to functional psychoses than the general population is inaccurate. Even patients with epilepsy who are diagnosed as psychotic usually have atypical patterns of intellectual and mood disorders [8]. Individuals with psychotic affective disorders rarely exhibit bipolar (manic-depressive) psychosis, a pattern that is fairly common in patients with functional affective psychoses [8]. Epileptic patients with the clinical features of schizophrenia are also different from nonepileptic schizophrenic patients in that they have less abnormal premorbid personalities, exhibit more paranoid delusions and ideas of reference, and are less likely to have catatonia associated with their thought disorders [8]. With both affective and cognitive disorders, the course of the disturbance in patients with epilepsy is much more variable than that in people with strictly functional disease [8].

The psychological disorders exhibited by patients with complex partial epilepsy range from hyperkinetic behavior and aggression to sexual dysfunction and hypochondriasis [10–13]. Signs and symptoms similar to those appearing in schizophrenia and psychotic depression do occur more commonly in patients with complex partial seizures than with any other type of seizure disorder, but truly psychotic symptoms are rare, though also more common than in patients with other types of epilepsy [10, 13, 14].

Complex partial seizures do not necessarily arise in the temporal lobe, but many do, and much of the psychopathology observed is associated with temporal lobe seizure foci. Obsessive and paranoid personality traits develop with uncommon frequency in individuals whose epileptic activity originates in the temporal lobe and who developed their seizures before puberty. These same individuals also exhibit a peculiar type of religious sentiment; some have multiple religious conversions, often reporting that a mystical experience was the basis for the conversion [13]. They are often paranoid, but their paranoia has a truly cosmic character: God or gods interact with them in fairly intimate ways. Commonplace events are filled with meaning [15]. A book will fall open with a passage warning them of their fate or pointing out the proper course to follow. Tragedies of all sorts are divine instructions. In some cultures, these individuals are considered devout; in others, they are dismissed as fanatics.

Another behavioral pattern that occurs with relatively high frequency in individuals with complex partial epilepsy is a compulsion to write. This hypergraphia may be limited to keeping very detailed diaries, or it may extend to spending much of the day writing. Inconsequential events will be recorded in extraordinary detail, but much of the material is redundant [15]. As with idiosyncratic religious behavior, this hypergraphia may be applauded in some social settings. Some successful writers have published more than 200 books during their adult life, and the written output of many academic physicians and research scientists has been no less substantial: This is legitimately considered hypergraphia, but it is not necessarily a pathologic personality trait.

Personality Changes

The personality changes that are described in individuals with a variety of seizure disorders, especially if the seizures develop after adolescence, often are neither pathologic nor undesirable. A routinely abusive man may mellow considerably after he develops complex partial seizures. An intractably shy woman may become more outgoing. These types of personality changes warrant no attention or intervention, but if the epileptic individual does become more violent or self-destructive, psychiatric intervention may be needed.

FEAR

In some individuals, especially those with seizure foci in the temporal lobe, overwhelming fear develops with the seizures or between seizure episodes [16]. If it is part of the ictus, it is called *ictal fear* [16]. This ictal fear is the commonest emotion felt by individuals with epilepsy during seizures, and it is reported in as many as 22 percent of individuals with temporal lobe seizure foci [16].

More difficult to understand is the appearance of a more abiding fear in many of these individuals, a fear that lasts for hours or days between the obvious seizure activity. Unlike ictal fear, which is prominent regardless of which temporal lobe has the seizure focus, this interictal fear, and particularly that which is specifically elicited by social and sexual experiences, is more likely to occur with a left-sided seizure focus than with a right-sided one [16]. That the type of interictal fear experienced by individuals with temporal lobe seizure foci is so specific supports the notion that it is fundamentally an expression of the epilepsy or the damage to the temporal lobe, rather than an affective response to the chronic menace of the seizure disorder.

This fear has some peculiar features. It does not involve a fear of injury or fear of animals, and men with right temporal lobe foci have less fear overall than men with left temporal lobe seizure foci [16]. The role that epilepsy actually plays in the appearance of this affective trait is uncertain. The seizure disorder may be an incidental finding in individuals with interictal fear and mood disturbances. Many of these patterns of fear appear in patients with brain damage not associated with epilepsy.

VIOLENT BEHAVIOR

The erroneous notion that people with epilepsy are routinely and unpredictably violent still persists in the nonmedical community, but it is more a worry than a belief for most people. Publicized accounts of people claiming to have committed violent crimes while unconscious or in a trance keep this fear alive. However, violent behavior is not common among average people with epilepsy. In the medical community, a very lively debate has long surrounded the question of violence in epilepsy. Some neurologists and neurosurgeons have argued that violent behavior is more frequent in specific types of epilepsy. Others do not find this pattern in their patients.

Reactive depressions and other common mood disturbances certainly do appear in epileptic patients at least as often as in individuals with other chronic diseases. Depression and anger are often appropriate reactions to poorly controlled epilepsy and unpleasant medications. Sometimes this depression fosters violence and destructive behavior that may not be obviously linked to the psychological problems. After all patients who might exhibit violent or aggressive behavior on these bases are excluded, there are still some patients with epilepsy who exhibit unexplained violent, aggressive, or sociopathic behavior. Much of this behavior is destructive; some of it is criminal. That epilepsy is responsible for any of it is controversial.

Family members are easy targets of violence when abusive behavior does occur in a person with seizures. Many of the injuries sustained by family members occur because they try to deal with the individual who is impaired by seizure activity as if that individual were rational and coherent. Although this abusive behavior is often an obvious part of the ictus, the aura, or the postictal period, some instances of abusive behavior occur long before or after seizure episodes. When the abusive behavior has no consistent provocation and the individuals most severely abused are those who are near at hand, seizure control should be considered an important factor in the behavior, and complete suppression of the seizures should be the principal objective of treatment.

Postictal Violence

Violence that occurs with postictal confusion is fairly common and largely innocuous. After the ictus, many patients injure themselves in confused efforts to resume normal activities. Some also exhibit an idiosyncratic hostility that may manifest itself as abusive language and defensive postures, which subside with the postictal confusion. Most epileptic individuals with this transient paranoid or aggressive behavior cause no damage to their surroundings and have little or no recall of the behavior after it abates [17]. Those who actually injure people around them usually do so while being restrained by well-intentioned bystanders [18]. Many patients try to get up or move about during the confusion that follows a generalized tonic-clonic seizure. If they are held down, they may strike out at the people trying to hold them and injure themselves or the other involved parties.

Ictal Violence

Aggressive behavior during a seizure is occasionally a reaction to delusions or hallucinations (Table 11–1). The current consensus among neurologists is that purposeful, violent behavior is not characteristic of any particular type of epilepsy [18, 19]. Purposeful aggression is never an ictal manifestation. An epileptic patient may damage property or injure people nearby who try to subdue him when he is confused or convulsing, but this violence is so obviously purposeless that only the most suspicious person will misconstrue

Table 11–1.
Ictal Violence

Abrupt appearance
Fragmented and unsustained
Purposeless
Lasts less than 1 minute
Stereotyped aggressive actions
Associated with automatisms
Nonspecific target
Expression suggests fear or anger

the damage as intentional [20]. Patients with auditory or visual hallucinations may react to threatening images or sounds with violent outbursts directed toward real people and objects.

Aggressive gestures, such as kicking, scratching, boxing, or spitting, appear in some individuals during the ictus of complex partial seizures. As a rule, this behavior appears abruptly and with no apparent planning. The behavior is stereotyped and appears with each fully developed seizure. If there is a target for the aggressive actions, such as a face to scratch or a person to kick, the target will be chosen indiscriminately. The aggressive behavior usually follows or occurs in conjunction with a variety of automatisms, including lip smacking, chewing, swallowing, and blinking [18].

None of the patients with ictal violence exhibit a period of staring or akinesia before the aggressive actions. If there is a change in facial expression associated with the violence, it generally suggests extreme fear or anger. Patients with kicking or boxing movements often shout in apparent fear and try to run away after their aggressive gestures. None of these patients with ictal violence makes any effort to conceal the aggressive acts, and no well-documented case of ictal violence has involved the acquisition and use of a weapon [18].

Ictal violence is an extremely fragmented and unsustained activity. It usually lasts approximately 30 seconds and never lasts more than 1 minute [18]. This ictal violence is much less common than postictal agitation, but it can be more dangerous. Fortunately, it generally is too random and disorganized to cause much real injury to anyone except the victim of the epilepsy.

Interictal Violence

Some of the sociopathic or violent behavior occurring in patients with epilepsy bears no relationship to seizure activity. Whether this violent behavior can be attributed to abnormal brain activity induced by the epilepsy or to intellectual and affective problems associated with brain damage is controversial. Rage and pointless hyperactivity are clearly more typical of diffuse brain damage than of diffuse seizure disorders [5]. Interictal violence and sociopathic behavior probably occur primarily in those epileptic individuals who have diffuse or strategically placed lesions in the brain.

Pleas in criminal courts that ascribe a defendant's actions to epilepsy have contributed most to the view that criminal activities can be the result of epileptic activity. Defense attorneys allege that the accused person apprehended after an aggressive, violent, or simply felonious activity was having a seizure at the time of the crime, and because of the temporary mental defect associated with the alleged seizure, the defendant cannot be held responsible for his criminal activities. Complex partial epilepsy is the favored diagnosis in pleading this defense, because its ictal and postictal manifestations are extremely diverse. Despite its popularity in court, most neurologists do not believe that repeated violence and destructive behavior can be ascribed to this type of epilepsy or any other type [11, 19, 21]. The prevalence of epilepsy among prison inmates, at least in England, is only slightly greater than that in the general population [19]. Individuals with epilepsy may commit robbery, assault, rape, or murder, but in these acts, their epilepsy is irrelevant.

Violence with Complex Partial Epilepsy

Violent behavior as a manifestation of complex partial epilepsy has been the subject of numerous studies, but the findings have been remarkably inconsistent [22]. Certain observations have been made repeatedly. There is a high incidence of sociopathy and psychopathology in patients followed in seizure disorder clinics for complex partial epilepsy from temporal lobe damage, but these clinic patients are highly selected [23]: They are usually indigent and have poor seizure control. As a group, they have many social problems.

Studies linking complex partial seizures with aggressive, destructive, or otherwise sociopathic behavior have been primarily preoperative or postoperative evaluations of epileptic patients subjected to surgery for relief of intractable seizures [22, 24]. In these patients, temporal lobe damage is found in 80 percent of cases, a high rate of pathologic change for any population of individuals with epilepsy [24]. Interictal aggressive behavior is the commonest psychological problem. Although children with temporal lobe epilepsy alone do not have unprovoked episodes of destructive behavior, the epileptic individuals most likely to exhibit irrational destructive or abusive behavior as adults are those whose seizures start in childhood [23, 24]. After the anterior temporal lobe is removed, the aggressive behavior remits for more than 6 years in 27 percent of the patients who undergo brain surgery [24].

Being male and having a low intelligence quotient, lack of religious ties, and a juvenile behavioral problem correlate better with the appearance of aggression in epileptic individuals than does the epilepsy itself [25, 26]. Forty-one percent of the patients who do exhibit aggressive behavior have faced permanent separation from one or both parents before they were 15 years old [25]. In many cases, it is violent behavior, rather than seizures, that initially prompts medical attention.

In children with complex partial epilepsy originating in the temporal lobes, episodes of minimally provoked rage and hyperactive behavior may develop when the seizures first appear [11]. Although such hyperkinetic behavior and rage occur less frequently as the individual with epilepsy ages, problems with recurrent depressions appear [11]. The adult with psychomotor epilepsy is often irritable and may have wide mood swings [27].

Probably most important in determining whether the individual with complex partial seizures will have violent or sociopathic outbursts is the type of damage that has occurred in the temporal lobe. The abnormal personality traits, change in personality, and seizure activity developing in these patients secondary to temporal lobe injury may all arise separately as a result of the structural damage to the brain.

Instances of violent or aggressive behavior appear in patients with types of epilepsy other than complex partial. Patients with generalized seizures who are young or who have myoclonic seizures are less likely to exhibit inappropriate aggression than older individuals with tonic-clonic seizures [22]. Individuals with akinetic seizures have a clearly increased incidence of violent behavior [22].

Children with complex partial epilepsy, focal motor or focal sensory epilepsy, or generalized tonic-clonic epilepsy are found to score at about the same levels on objective ratings of aggression, social competence, and overall behavior dysfunction [26]. There is no significant difference in the aggression scores of the population with complex partial epilepsy and those with generalized tonic-clonic seizures, which indicates that the problem of violence is not substantial in or peculiar to the group of patients with complex partial epilepsy.

Violence with Improved Seizure Control

In some cases, violent behavior becomes more prominent as the epilepsy is better controlled. Some patients with complex partial epilepsy have frequent violent outbursts during long seizure-free intervals [11]. The abusive behavior may last hours to days and stop abruptly when a seizure occurs. During the irritable interictal period, the patients resists all efforts to calm him and broods over imagined slights and insults. There is little real chance that such an impaired patient will cause injury to people trying to reason with him; and, when the anger abates, the patient usually is remorseful and apologetic [11]. He remembers the behavior but cannot explain what prompted it.

Increasing control of the seizures may increase the frequency of the episodes. Consequently, some clinicians allow their patients to remain incompletely controlled if violent behavior is an interictal problem [11]. Allowing seizures to recur carries its own risks, because injury or status epilepticus may result. If the violence poses a real threat to the patient himself or to those around him, antipsychotic medication may be helpful, even though many of these drugs lower the seizure threshold slightly. Achieving full control of the epilepsy should remain the clinician's objective, because when seizures no longer occur at all, the worsening violent behavior may abate completely.

It is well established that much of the violence observed in individuals with seizures that originate in the temporal lobes abates after surgery. Some physicians have used this fact to justify performing a temporal lobe operation to control violent behavior itself, but the long-term effects of the operation are too controversial and the basis for the observed changes is too poorly understood to recommend a surgical approach to managing violent behavior in individuals with or without epilepsy. The advantages and disadvantages of operating on the brain as a treatment for refractory seizures is discussed in Chapter 15.

EPISODIC DYSCONTROL

Although epilepsy plays a negligible role in sociopathic and criminal behavior, there clearly is a disorganized emotional or intellectual state involved in many violent acts. To minimize the arguments about whether this is a voluntary or involuntary condition, it has been called the *episodic dyscontrol syndrome,* a term that avoids any inference about the basis for the condition [28]. People with this syndrome have bouts of violent behavior that last minutes to hours. These outbursts usually are unprovoked, and some of the people who exhibit them claim they are preceded by abnormal sensations. After the violence, most individuals with this syndrome have considerable fatigue or headache.

The grouping of these behavioral disorders into a syndrome implies that a nervous system disorder may underlie the violence [21]. Epilepsy probably is not responsible for this pattern of sociopathic behavior, but the responsible agent, other than a personality disorder, remains undetermined. Half of the individuals with this syndrome claim to have experienced staring spells, unrelated to violent behavior, with several seconds of "altered consciousness" [28]. Alcohol use increases the frequency and severity of the violent episodes. People with this type of behavior often claim that just before the violence they had visual illusions, altered hearing, nausea, or paresthesias [28]. After the attack, they often deny all recall of the episode or claim that they were not in control of their own behavior.

These features of episodic dyscontrol are no more suggestive of epilepsy than they are of extreme excitement or agitation. Seventy-two percent of violent juvenile offenders claim memory lapses, blackouts, dizziness, and dream-like states during the crime and excessive fatigue afterward [21]. Many of the personality traits of the affected individuals suggest more a psychological problem than a neurologic one. People with this syndrome generally are men, usually from poor families [28]. They invariably have little formal education and exhibit sociopathic behavior by the time they are 20 or 30 years old. Their fathers often are chronic alcoholics, and family histories routinely show a recurrent pattern of child abuse. More than 70 percent of the men with episodic dyscontrol as adults were hyperactive as children [28]. Most claim that they regret the violent behavior that brought them to medical or judicial attention, and approximately 50 percent report having attempted suicide at some time [28]. More than 30 percent admit to sexual problems or idiosyncracies, such as impotence, transvestism, and obsessive abstinence from sex [29].

One bit of evidence which supports the notion that episodic dyscontrol is at least distantly related to epilepsy is the apparent beneficial effect of anti-epileptic drugs in these individuals [28]. Sixty-eight percent of men with episodic dyscontrol syndrome exhibit fewer violent outbursts when they take phenytoin [28]. That this improvement is actually related to the drug's antiepileptic effect is unknown. If these men are given no treatment, the syndrome still disappears after several years, a not surprising finding since most types of sociopathic and violent behavior are less common in older men. Episodic dyscontrol rarely persists after 50 years of age and usually remits long before this [28].

Objective study of these violent individuals is very difficult. Evidence collected for court hearings is far from impartial. Individuals alleged to have the syndrome have a great deal to gain by convincing judicial officials that the underlying problem is a seizure disorder. This questionable evidence may account for some of the studies which report an incidence of epilepsy in prison populations that is ten times that seen in the general population [17, 29].

FUGUE STATES

With some types of seizures, the patient may have very long seizure episodes during which he or she enters a trance-like state. This is most common with generalized absence (petit mal) and complex partial seizures, but it is exceedingly rare in both. These are called *fugue states,* a term more commonly used to refer to protracted episodes of confused activity seen in individuals with schizophrenia or other psychoses. Patients with fugue states caused by seizure activity are usually much less active and independent than patients with schizophrenic episodes [7].

The fugue state usually is a nonconvulsive status epilepticus, but because it goes on for many hours or days, during which the patient exhibits considerable activity, it is described as a distinct entity. By designating a condition as a fugue state, the physician simply states his or her inability to determine whether the patient is having continuous nonconvulsive seizure activity, frequently recurrent seizures with postictal confusion, or merely protracted postictal confusion. Activity during the fugue state is highly disorganized and largely purposeless. The patient may be able to survive in this state for several days without much assistance, but he cannot commit a crime or perform any but the most familiar tasks.

Some patients with typical fugue states are described as being in an epileptic twilight state, but this is inaccurate. The *twilight state* classically refers to a protracted interval of confused behavior following nonconvulsive status epilepticus [30]. The distinction between the fugue state and the twilight state may be very difficult to make. During the epileptic twilight state, the patient should not have demonstrable seizure activity, but the electroencephalogram usually will be abnormal. After the episode, the patient generally will not recall what transpired and may actually have a memory impairment that persists for days or weeks after the resolution of the twilight state [30]. Unlike the individual who claims to have had a period of amnesia during which he robbed a bank or killed his wife's lover, the individual in an epileptic twilight state will not be able to perform complex activities.

SUICIDE

Suicide and nonindustrial accidents are relatively common causes of death for patients with epilepsy. Self-destructive behavior exhibited by these patients ranges from inadvisable risk taking to unequivocal suicide attempts. It may derive from the depression that often accompanies any chronic medical problem, but with some types of epilepsy, the seizure disorder itself seems to contribute to the affective disturbance that increases the incidence of self-destructive behavior. Individuals with complex partial epilepsy, in particular, have mood disturbances that dispose them to suicidal activities, and patients with most types of epilepsy have access to medications that can painlessly endanger their lives [12]. Many suicide attempts clearly are little more than gestures fostered by frustration, but even when the gesture is ambivalent, the outcome may be lethal.

In many cases, accidental deaths are caused in part by patient negligence or indifference. Many patients told they should not drive still do. Driving an automobile when seizure control is poor is always dangerous, but it is even riskier when there have been recent changes in antiepileptic drug dosages that can slow reaction times. These facts are obvious to any person intact enough to drive a motor vehicle, and so those who disregard the dangers they face must be indifferent to the outcome or must strenuously deny the risk.

Mood Disturbances

The incidence of depressive disorders has changed very little over the past 30 years, despite substantial advances in seizure control. Serious mood disturbances are not limited to individuals who require hospitalization or institutionalization for frequent seizures [11]. Seventeen to 25 percent of epileptic patients who are not institutionalized or hospitalized have psychiatric problems that interfere with their ability to function normally, and at least 10 percent have problems severe enough to necessitate psychiatric hospitalization [11]. A suicide attempt is often the reason for that hospitalization. The individuals who have the most severe mood disturbances frequently are much less disabled than people with other chronic problems who exhibit no affective disorders [31]. The severity of the depression does not parallel the severity of the epilepsy.

Damage to the left hemisphere of the brain typically increases the depressive episodes to which the individual is subject [32]. Unexplained bouts of crying may develop with left hemisphere disease, and unprovoked laughing may be seen in individuals with right hemisphere lesions [16]. The practical implication of this is that mood disorders in individuals with seizure disorders might be better approached through treatment with mood-altering drugs than through drug-free psychotherapy.

Suicide Attempts

Attempted suicide is common among patients with all types of epilepsy [12, 33]. Along with lethal events that are a direct expression of the epilepsy, such as status epilepticus and seizure-related accidents, suicide ranks as a leading cause of death in individuals with seizures [33]. The prominence of suicide as a cause of death is evident even without making adjustments for probable suicides. As in any population of patients, there is a group in which the cause of death appears to be accidental or is never defined as anything more than an unexplained cardiac arrest. Many of these probably are suicides [34].

As many as 12 to 20 percent of deaths in individuals with epilepsy are caused by suicide [34–37]. The prevalence of suicidal individuals in the population with epilepsy is 32.5 per 1,000 [12]. This is five times the prevalence of individuals attempting suicide in the general population [33]. The group at highest risk is that with complex partial epilepsy. The rate of suicide attempts in this group may be as much as twenty-five times greater than that of the general population [33].

Eighty-four percent of epileptic individuals who attempt suicide use self-poisoning, and in 65 percent of these instances, the agents are antiepileptic drugs [12, 37]. Phenobarbital has always been especially popular in suicide attempts by epileptic patients [12]. The respiratory depressant action of this drug often is purposely enhanced by alcohol abuse coinciding with the drug overdose. Approximately two-thirds of the epileptic individuals who poison themselves take an anticonvulsant they have been prescribed, and another 15 percent combine their anticonvulsants with other drugs [38].

Even though phenobarbital is being supplanted by other anticonvulsants, many of the antiepileptic medications in use are either metabolized to phenobarbital or can depress breathing even though they are not barbiturates. With closer supervision of medication by the physician, the suicide rate is lower. Patients in hospitals or other institutions are much less likely to commit suicide than epileptic individuals who are living outside such facilities [37].

Epileptic men more often attempt suicide than epileptic women, but both men and women are more inclined to attempt suicide when they are unemployed [12]. This is not a response to decades of problems with seizure control and social maladjustment: Suicide occurs primarily in young people. Sixty percent of the people with epilepsy who attempt suicide are younger than 30 years [12]. Most attempts at self-destruction are sincere rather than just provocative gestures to attract attention or help for emotional problems. Repeated suicide attempts are twice as common in people with epilepsy as in people without epilepsy: 74 percent of epileptic patients who attempt suicide and fail will try again [37, 38].

If suicide attempts fail, it is often because the patient is misinformed or has misconceptions; what he believes to be lethal may be fairly innocuous. The individual on phenytoin may take a massive dose in an obvious suicide attempt and suffer little more than protracted gait difficulty, blurred vision, nausea, and vomiting. Obviously, the patient at greatest risk of repeated suicide attempts is the one who fails through misinformation alone. Careful observation and aggressive treatment of these individuals is important in any plan to avert a successful suicide.

All efforts to reduce the risk of future suicide attempts must take into consideration the events leading to the self-destructive action. Multiple problems usually contribute to the individual's sense of hopelessness, but there is often a single incident or unresolvable problem that triggers the final gesture at self-extinction. Some people ascribe their despair to profound guilt over being constantly dependent. Problems with seizure control often are cited as justification for the suicide attempts, but the true basis for the self-destructive behavior may be more subtle. A spouse's abuse, prompted by financial worries or problems with seizure control, may be more instrumental in precipitating a suicide attempt than unemployment or epilepsy [38].

Noncompliance

Major psychiatric disorders, such as schizophrenia and manic-depressive psychoses, are no more common in individuals with epilepsy who make suicide attempts than in people without seizure disorders who try to kill or injure themselves, but there is a higher incidence of personality disorders among suicidal individuals with epilepsy [38]. Patients with epilepsy face social problems because of their chronic disorder. In addition, they are burdened with personality disorders that often limit their ability to manage the problems they face.

The patient's psychological problems may frustrate all efforts to effectively control seizures. Poor compliance with the recommended medication regimen is the commonest basis for recurrent seizures in a previously well-controlled patient. The patient's decision to stop the use of all antiepileptics may precipitate status epilepticus. Although this behavior generally is not included in statistics on suicidal gestures, it probably accounts for as much morbidity and mortality as frank suicide attempts.

An equally dangerous option available to the person with seizures is noncompliance with restrictions on activity. Swimming, driving, rock climbing, and commuting by subway can all pose substantial threats to the individual whose seizures are poorly controlled.

TREATING DEPRESSION

If the patient is profoundly depressed, antidepressant medication may be appropriate on a short-term basis to minimize the risk of repeated suicide attempts. In many cases, psychotherapy on an individual or group basis may be more important than medication in helping the patient manage the problems that precipitated a suicide attempt, but treatment of the severely depressed person with epilepsy must be intensive and carefully conceived. No patient should be left unsupervised or untreated simply because he insists that he feels fine and does not need help.

Antidepressant Medication

In many cases, successful therapy requires antidepressant medication, but treating mood disturbances with psychotropic drugs presents special problems for the person with epilepsy. Many antidepressants, such as the tricyclic compounds imipramine hydrochloride (Tofranil), amitriptyline hydrochloride (Elavil), and nortriptyline hydrochloride, lower the seizure threshold and may induce seizures at toxic levels. These are particularly dangerous for depressed patients who might ignore instructions on how to take the drugs [39, 40]. Some physicians recommend using maprotiline (Desyrel) because of its lower incidence of associated seizures, but the risk of inducing seizures with any of these antidepressants is fairly low at therapeutic dosages [39]. The risk of increased seizure activity is actually greater with maprotiline than with the tricyclic compounds if the patient takes a substantial overdose [39].

Doxepin hydrochloride is the least likely of any of the commonly used antidepressants to induce seizures, but it generally is not as effective an antidepressant as the other more provocative drugs. There are some antidepressants that are not widely used, such as viloxazine hydrochloride, which may actually reduce seizure frequency when given in therapeutic doses [39]. The selection of the drug to be used must be based on both the patient's susceptibility to seizures and the probable efficacy of the antidepressant.

Treating the patient with neuroleptics, whether they are phenothiazines or butyrophenones, carries little risk of increasing the seizure frequency [39]. Some patients with affective disorders may respond well to these drugs, and the risks associated with an intentional overdose are substantially lower than with antidepressants [40]. Poisoning with an antidepressant will typically cause seizures in approximately 12 percent of patients taking the most commonly prescribed antidepressants, whereas poisoning with a neuroleptic causes seizures in only about 7 percent [39].

Electroconvulsive Therapy

In cases of severe depression in nonepileptic patients, the physician has the option of using electroconvulsive therapy [41]. However, such therapy is more dangerous than tricyclic antidepressants or neuroleptics in epileptic patients, because it induces a seizure. Initiating a seizure in a patient with epilepsy exposes him to an increased risk of status epilepticus or other complications of seizure activity. Of course, the highly controlled nature of electroshock therapy, when properly applied, minimizes these risks, but it cannot eliminate them [41]. If the patient is having generalized seizures at the time of the severe depression, it is unlikely that electroshock therapy, which will simply increase the patient's number of seizures per week, will have much impact on the affective disorder. This does not mean that treatment of the depression, anxiety, or fear experienced by these individuals is inadvisable: what it does mean is that drug regimens and electroconvulsive shock must be applied with attention to the risks of increased seizure frequency.

Minimizing Self-Destructive Behavior

Much of the self-destructive behavior exhibited by depressed patients with epilepsy can be eliminated with close patient follow-up. The physician cannot assume that the patient who is well controlled and in good spirits will continue in this state. Periodic visits (every 6 months) will allow reassessment of the patient who is doing well, and more frequent visits will allow early recognition of depressive symptoms in patients who are having more seizures. If the patient has had an increasing number of accidents, the physician may legitimately recommend that he be hospitalized and that a psychiatrist be involved in the assessment of the patient. Unfortunately, most patients will resist this suggestion, and it is up to the physician primarily responsible for the patient to try to introduce psychotropic agents to manage the patient's depression on a short-term basis. Continuing management of the depressive disorder may also fall to the primary physician, but more intensive psychiatric attention should be urged at each follow-up visit.

REFERENCES

1. Dodrill, C.B., Batzel, L.W., Queisser, H.R., et al. An objective method for the assessment of psychological and social problems among epileptics. *Epilepsia* 21:123–135, 1980.
2. Ryan, R., Kempner, K., Emlen, A.C. The stigma of epilepsy as a self-concept. *Epilepsia* 21:433–444, 1980.
3. Stevens, J.R. Psychosis and epilepsy. *Ann. Neurol.* 14(3):347–348, 1983.
4. Hermann, B.P., Schwartz, M.S., Karnes, W.E., et al. Psychopathology in epilepsy: relationship of seizure type to age at onset. *Epilepsia* 21:15–23, 1980.
5. Camfield, P.R., Gates, R., Ronen, G., et al. Comparison of cognitive ability, personality profile, and school success in epileptic children with pure right versus left temporal lobe EEG foci. *Ann. Neurol.* 15(2):122–126, 1984.
6. Lund, M., Reintoft, H., Simonsen, N. En kontrollerot social og psykologisk undersogelse af patienter med juvenil myoklon epilepsi. *Ugeskr. Laeger* 137:2415–2418, 1975.

7. Lechtenberg, R. *The Psychiatrist's Guide to Diseases of The Nervous System.* New York: John Wiley & Sons, 1982.
8. Toone, B.K., Garralda, M.E., Ron, M.A. The psychoses of epilepsy and the functional psychoses: a clinical and phenomenological comparison. *Br. J. Psychiatry* 141:256–261, 1982.
9. Mayeux, R., Brandt, J., Rosen, J., et al. Interictal memory and language impairment in temporal lobe epilepsy. *Neurology* (N.Y.) 10:120, 1980.
10. Bear, D.M., Fedio, P. Quantitative analysis of interictal behavior in temporal lobe epilepsy. *Arch. Neurol.* 32:454, 1977.
11. Blumer, D. Temporal lobe epilepsy and its psychiatric significance. In Benson, D.F., Blumer, D. (eds.), *Psychiatric Aspects of Neurologic Disease.* New York: Grune & Stratton, 1975, p. 171.
12. Hawton, K., Fagg, J., Marsack, P. Association between epilepsy and attempted suicide. *J. Neurol. Neurosurg. Psychiatry* 43:168, 1980.
13. Slater, E., Beard, A.W. The schizophrenia-like psychoses of epilepsy. Psychiatric aspects. *Br. J. Psychiatry* 109:95, 1963.
14. Serafetinides, E.A. Aggressiveness in temporal lobe epileptics and its relation to cerebral dysfunction and environmental factors. *Epilepsia* 6:33, 1965.
15. Valenstein, E., Heilman, K.M. Emotional disorders resulting from lesions of the central nervous system. In Heilman, K.M., Valenstein, E. (eds.), *Clinical Neuropsychology.* New York: Oxford University Press, 1979, p. 413.
16. Strauss, E., Risser, A., Jones, M.W. Fear responses in patients with epilepsy. *Arch. Neurol.* 39(10):626–630, 1982.
17. Goldstein, M. Brain research and violent behavior. *Arch. Neurol.* 30:1, 1974.
18. Delgado-Escueta, A.V., Mattson, R., King, L., et al. The nature of aggression during epileptic seizures. *N. Engl. J. Med.* 305(12):711–716, 1981.
19. Gunn, J. Violence and epilepsy. *N. Engl. J. Med.* 306:298–299, 1982.
20. Poeck, K. Pathophysiology of emotional disorders associated with brain damage. In Vinken, P.J., Bruyn, G.W. (eds.), *Handbook of Clinical Neurology,* vol. 3. New York: American Elsevier Publishing Co., 1969, p. 343.
21. Pincus, J.H. Can violence be a manifestation of epilepsy? *Neurology* (N.Y.) 30:304, 1980.
22. Hermann, B.P., Schwartz, M.S., Whitman, S., et al. Aggression and epilepsy: seizure-type comparisons and high-risk variables. *Epilepsia* 21:691–698, 1980.
23. Stevens, J.R. Interictal clinical manifestations of complex partial seizures. *Adv. Neurol.* 11:85, 1975.
24. Falconer, M.A. Reversibility by temporal-lobe resection of the behavioral abnormalities of temporal-lobe epilepsy. *N. Engl. J. Med.* 289:451, 1973.
25. Taylor, D.C. Aggression and epilepsy. *J. Psychosom. Res.* 13:229, 1969.
26. Hermann, B.P., Black, R.B., Chhabria, S. Behavioral problems and social competence in children with epilepsy. *Epilepsia* 22:703–710, 1981.
27. Rodin, E.A. Psychosocial management of patients with complex partial seizures. *Adv. Neurol.* 11:383; 1975.
28. Maletzky, B.M. The episodic dyscontrol syndrome. *Dis. Nerv. Syst.* 34:178, 1973.
29. Bach-Y-Rita, G., Lion, J.R., Climent, C.E., et al. Episodic dyscontrol: a study of 130 violent patients. *Am. J. Psychiatry* 127:1473, 1971.
30. Ballenger, C.E., III, King, D.W., Gallagher, B.B. Partial complex status epilepticus. *Neurology* (N.Y.) 33(12):1545–1552, 1983.
31. Bracht, N.F. The social nature of chronic disease and disability. *Soc. Work Health Care* 5(2):129–144, 1979.
32. Brooks, D.N., Aughton, M.E., Bond, M.R., et al. Cognitive sequelae in relationship to early indices of severity of brain damage after severe blunt head injury. *J. Neurol. Neurosurg. Psychiatry* 43:529, 1980.

33. Barraclough, B.   Suicide and epilepsy. In Reynolds, E.H., Trimble, M.R. (eds.), *Epilepsy and Psychiatry.* New York: Churchill Livingstone, 1981, pp. 72–76.
34. Woodbury, L.A.   Shortening of the lifespan and mortality of patients with epilepsy. In The Commission for the Control of Epilepsy and Its Consequences, *Plan for Nationwide Action on Epilepsy,* vol. 4. Washington, D.C.: U.S. Department of Health, Education and Welfare, 1978.
35. Zielinski, J.J.   Epilepsy and mortality rate and cause of death. *Epilepsia* 16:191–201, 1974.
36. Hauser, W.A., Annegers, J.F., Elveback, L.R.   Mortality in patients with epilepsy. *Epilepsia* 21:399–412, 1980.
37. Matthews, W.S., Barabas, M.   Suicide and epilepsy: a review of the literature. *Psychosomatics* 22(6):515–524, 1981.
38. Mackay, A.   Self-poisoning—a complication of epilepsy. *Br. J. Psychiatry* 134:277–282, 1979.
39. Luchina, D.J., Oliver, A.P., Wyatt, R.J.   Seizures with antidepressants: an in vitro technique to assess relative risk. *Epilepsia* 25(1):25–32, 1984.
40. Shopsin, B., Waters, B.   The pharmacotherapy of major depressive syndrome: 1: Treatment of acute depression. *Psychosomatics* 21:542, 1980.
41. Blackwood, D.H.R., Cull, R.E., Freeman, C.P.L., et al.   A study of the incidence of epilepsy following ECT. *J. Neurol. Neurosurg. Psychiatry* 43:1098, 1980.

12. Treatment Principles

Most types of epilepsy can be managed with antiepileptic drugs alone. In every case of well-established epilepsy, drugs should be the first type of treatment used. Alternatives, such as dietary manipulation, surgery, biofeedback, and less conventional techniques, should only be tried after antiepileptic drugs have clearly failed. Even when alternatives are used, the antiepileptics should be continued until the patient is seizure-free. At that point, medications can be withdrawn cautiously.

Which medication should be used first is determined by several factors. The age of the patient, the type and severity of the epilepsy, and the patient's prior experience with antiepileptic drugs all influence the decision. Whenever any drug is used, it is best to start with only one drug [1]. If one drug fails, other drugs should be tried individually until all reasonable choices have been exhausted. If a single drug cannot be found that will completely suppress the epilepsy, then using two or more antiepileptic drugs in combination may prove effective.

Of course, there are seizure disorders that can be controlled without antiepileptic drugs. Correctable metabolic problems, such as hypoglycemia or hypocalcemia, are best managed by achieving normal glucose or calcium levels. If the seizure was induced by a specific stimulus, then avoiding future seizures may require simply avoidance of the provocative stimulus. With an electrical shock, the seizure may recur only with another shock. Unfortunately, most causes of seizures are not so easily remedied, and the victim of the epilepsy is obliged to take medication for years or for life.

For each type of epilepsy, there is a medication that is considered the drug of choice. That drug is the one having the fewest adverse effects and the greatest efficacy for the majority of patients with that seizure disorder. Any drug used for an individual must consider that person's special problems. Someone allergic to carbamazepine cannot reasonably be treated with that drug, regardless of how well controlled his seizures are on that antiepileptic. Someone who has been seizure-free on an antiepileptic that is not usually effective against the type of seizure that he exhibits should be continued on that drug.

The drug of choice in any given case is based on a consensus, and that consensus changes frequently. Some epileptologists believed until recently that valproic acid should be considered the drug of choice for generalized tonic-clonic seizures, but this enthusiasm abated when reports of occasional hepatic problems induced by the drug began emerging [1]. Acetazolamide, a diuretic that inhibits carbonic anhydrase, was once considered the drug of choice for management of generalized absence seizures [2]. Currently, most physicians do not use this drug for the management of any type of epilepsy.

Even with the most appropriate treatment available, some patients continue to have seizures. Those who have persistently poor seizure control despite appropriate modifications in their life-styles, medication regimens, and level of cooperation may have a progressive central nervous system disease, fac-titious seizures, or a static brain lesion that is insensitive to antiepileptic drugs. The proper approach to each of these possibilities is very different, and so the physician's first responsibility is to ascertain the basis for the persistent seizures. Patients with authentic seizures from a static lesion may profit from surgery if the lesion is in an accessible region of the brain.

Occasionally, a patient will have seizures after several years of excellent control on medication. When seizures recur in this way, the problem is usually a change in the individual's life-style, general health, or level of compliance. Making adjustments for these changes will reestablish good seizure control in most cases.

TREATMENT GOALS

Regardless of the type of epilepsy the patient has, the treatment goal is to eliminate seizures without unduly disturbing the individual's life (Table 12–1). The epilepsy should not be the focus of the patient's energy and activity, and the antiepileptic medication should impose no additional burdens of its own. Ideally, the treatment should cure the problem. Currently, there are no antiepileptic drugs that will predictably eradicate epilepsy. Some drugs appear to increase the rate of remission with some types of epilepsy, but how in-

Table 12–1.
Outlook For Complete Seizure Control

Good	Poor
Strictly generalized seizures	Complex partial seizures with tonic-clonic activity as well
Strictly complex partial seizures	
Idiopathic basis for seizures	Seizures from tumor, stroke, contusion, meningitis, etc.
No intellectual impairment	
No personality disorder	Low I.Q.
Normal EEG or minor background abnormalities	Obvious personality disorder
	Anterior temporal or frontal lobe abnormalities on EEG
Treatment begun within 1 year of seizure onset	Treatment delayed
Onset of epilepsy at 2 to 5 years of age	Onset of epilepsy before 1 year of age

strumental the drugs are in actually eliminating the risk of seizures is controversial. With some types of epilepsy, the seizures remit spontaneously as the individual ages. In such cases, a fairly normal life can be achieved with any drug that will suppress the seizure activity until the individual's maturation eliminates the problem.

DRUGS OF CHOICE

Any physician managing a patient with epilepsy must be familiar with the drugs he or she is giving the patient. This means that the drug of choice will necessarily be influenced by each physician's experience, and this is amply reflected in the conflicting opinions among epileptologists and neurologists regarding which drug should be used for each type of epilepsy (Table 12–2). Most agree that phenytoin sodium (Dilantin) is still the most effective and

Table 12–2.
Drugs of Choice

Seizure Type	Anticonvulsant	
	Primary	Alternatives
Generalized tonic-clonic	Phenytoin	Valproic acid, carbamazepine, primidone, phenobarbital
Complex partial	Carbamazepine	Primidone
Generalized absence (petit mal, nonconvulsive)	Ethosuximide	Methsuximide, valproic acid, trimethadione
Simple partial	Phenytoin	Primidone
Benign juvenile myoclonic	Valproic acid	Ethosuximide, clonazepam, phenytoin
Complex febrile	Phenobarbital	Valproic acid, primidone
Rolandic	Valproic acid	Phenytoin
Idiopathic neonatal	Phenobarbital	Phenytoin, diazepam
Infantile spasms	Adrenocorticotropic hormone	Valproic acid, phenobarbital

safest drug available for treating generalized tonic-clonic seizures. Valproic acid (valproate sodium; Depakene) is also a very effective drug for this type of epilepsy and will probably be the drug of choice if experience demonstrates that it is safe.

Carbamazepine (Tegretol) is the first choice of many physicians for complex partial seizures. However, when it was initially introduced for management of this type of epilepsy, scattered reports of lethal thrombocytopenia associated with the drug tempered its popularity. Experience revealed that these were fairly rare idiosyncratic reactions and that attention to the patient's platelet count and white blood cell count could minimize the risk to the patient. Primidone (Mysoline) is still the best drug for managing complex partial seizures, as far as some physicians are concerned, and there is no argument that it is a valuable alternative to carbamazepine if that drug fails to control this type of seizure activity.

Generalized absence seizures are best managed with ethosuximide (Zarontin) or methsuximide (Celontin), and focal motor and focal sensory seizures respond best to phenytoin. Pediatricians prefer phenobarbital for complex febrile seizures, but valproic acid or phenytoin may soon replace this drug as the favored treatment when more experience is gained with these drugs in infants.

Every physician must consider the individual being treated when deciding the drug of choice. A young woman of childbearing age is likely to be concerned about the cosmetic, as well as the teratogenic, effects of any drug prescribed for management of her seizures. Even if she has generalized tonic-clonic seizures, she may be reluctant to use phenytoin because of the gingival hyperplasia and risk of fetal deformity associated with this drug. Obviously, this patient will be more compliant with an alternative drug, such as valproic acid. Young children may have severe gastrointestinal reactions to carbamazepine at very low doses. If the child has a history of frequent episodes of vomiting or diarrhea already, it would be better to start with primidone in efforts to manage complex partial seizures. The true drug of choice will vary from patient to patient.

Initiation of Treatment

Initially, every patient should be given only one antiepileptic medication [3]. The starting dose of most antiepileptic drugs usually is less than the daily dose that the patient ultimately will need to maintain a steady level of it in the blood. This may not be true if the patient has been on the antiepileptics before, in which case the plasma clearance of the drug will be higher than for the patient with no prior exposure to the drug [1].

To avoid sedation and gastrointestinal discomfort, the initial daily dose of carbamazepine or primidone should be one-third to one-fourth of the maintenance dose [1]. Starting at a full maintenance dose of valproic acid usually will produce nausea and vomiting. If the initial dose of any of these drugs causes no problems, it can be doubled within a day or two. If the patient tolerates the drug poorly, several weeks may be required to reach a maintenance dose. The amount of time required for the patient to tolerate the drug is influenced in large part by how quickly liver enzymes reponsible for metabolizing the drug are induced [1].

A notable exception to this approach for starting anticonvulsant drugs is phenytoin. A loading dose of 900 mg (for an adult) can be given in two or three doses on the first day of treatment, and a maintenance dose can usually be given on the second day [1]. The serum level of this drug rises very gradually, and so most toxic effects are not apparent until the drug has been given in excess for several days or weeks. Individuals especially sensitive to phenytoin may feel tired, stagger, slur their words, and complain of blurred vision after the loading dose, but most develop these toxic signs only after 1 or 2 weeks of excessive medication.

Surveillance of Effectiveness

The serum concentrations of all the drugs currently used as antiepileptics can be measured with widely available blood tests (Table 12–3). The dose required by a particular individual with seizures to maintain a therapeutic drug level in the serum can be measured precisely by periodic checking of the serum level. How often the drug level should be checked depends on the speed with which the drug is metabolized. A clonazepam level may be checked after a few days of use, whereas a phenytoin level will not show much change until after a week of a constant dosage. The best time of day to check a serum drug level is at the end of a dose interval—that is, just before the patient is about to take another dose of the drug to be measured [1].

If the drug is at a therapeutic serum level and the patient still is having seizures, then the effectiveness of the drug must be questioned. Before the drug is changed, it is wise to increase the daily dose to see if a slightly higher

Table 12–3.
Therapeutic Levels of Currently Popular Antiepileptics

Drug	Serum Levels (µg drug/ml serum)	Starting Dose (mg)	Daily Dose (mg)
Phenytoin	10–20	900 (15 mg/kg)	300–400
Carbamazepine	6–10	100–200	600–1,200
Valproic acid	50–100	250 (50–100)*	1,000–3,000
Ethosuximide	50–100	250	750–2,000
Primidone	6–12	50–125	750–1,500
Phenobarbital	15–35	30–60	100–150
Clonazepam	0.013–0.072	0.5	1–2

* For children.

serum level will be effective without being toxic [1]. If this, too, fails, then the patient probably needs a different anticonvulsant. The alternative is that the patient has factitious seizures and that no amount of anticonvulsant will suppress the seizure activity. If the physician is confident that the patient has epilepsy, then alternative drugs should be tried.

Any drug that is going to be effective is likely to be effective alone, but occasionally, a combination of two or more antiepileptics will be needed to suppress seizure activity. The combinations needed in an individual patient are determined by trial and error with drugs that have demonstrated efficacy against the type of seizures being treated and that the patient can tolerate.

Occasionally, the timing of the doses is as important as the total daily dose of the drug. Drugs with fairly rapid turnovers, like carbamazepine and primidone, may produce better results when given as several doses a few hours apart during the day. Although the serum level of the drug may increase only slightly or not at all, in such a regimen, the effectiveness of the drug may increase substantially because of less variation in the serum level between doses.

Surveillance of Compliance

Occasionally a patient fails to respond to antiepileptic treatment and fails to achieve substantial serum levels of the antiepileptic drug despite the administration of large doses. This may indicate poor drug compliance: The person with epilepsy is not taking the medication. Alternatively, the patient may be taking another drug that is interfering with the absorption or increasing the breakdown of the antiepileptic drug.

All possible drug interactions should be considered before it is assumed that the patient is not taking the drug. This is especially true when the patient is taking a combination of antiepileptics (Table 12–4). Either phenytoin or phenobarbital will increase the metabolism of carbamazepine and consequently reduce its serum half-life [1]. Warfarin sodium and other drugs that

Table 12–4.
Antiepileptic Drug Interactions

	Medication					
Action	PBA	VPA	PHT	CNP	CBZ	PMD
Serum level decreased by:	CBZ	PHT, PBA, CBZ, PMD	CBZ, VPA	CBZ, PHT, PBA	PHT, VPA, PBA	
Serum level increased by:	PHT, VPA		ETH			VPA

PBA = phenobarbital; VPA = valproic acid; PHT = phenytoin; CNP = clonazepam; CBZ = carbamazepine; PMD = primidone; ETH = ethosuximide.

induce hepatic enzymes can also speed up the metabolism of some anticonvulsants.

If poor compliance is likely, seizure control may be improved by admitting the patient to a hospital for better regulation of his or her medication. If the serum level of the drug increases while the patient is given the drug under rigorous supervision, it is reasonable to ask what the problem at home is. The patient may miss his medication doses because seizure activity interferes with his memory. He may believe that he takes the medication but actually forgets on a regular basis. If the patient willfully avoids taking the medication, then the reason for this behavior must be ascertained and addressed.

CONTROL OF SEIZURES WITH TREATMENT

How well an individual responds to medication is affected by the type of central nervous system problem causing the epilepsy, coincidental non-neurologic problems, and the patient's ability to absorb and metabolize the drug [4]. Patients responding best to drugs are those who have idiopathic epilepsies [5]. Even when there is an obvious basis for the seizure disorder, such as brain damage from head trauma or meningitis, the less frequent the seizure episodes are, the better the level of control that can be achieved [4].

The patient's age also affects the likelihood that complete seizure control will be achieved with medication alone. Seizures in patients who developed epilepsy before 10 years of age are generally more easily controlled than those in individuals who were older at seizure onset [5]. Good seizure control is most easily realized in patients starting on drugs within 1 year of their first seizure [6]. Epilepsy treated early and aggressively is less likely to be a chronic problem than epilepsy left untreated for months or years [3]. Eighty-seven percent of patients who are seizure-free during their first year of treatment will remain seizure-free for 3 years if they continue the treatment [1].

There are complications that interfere with even the most carefully fashioned treatment regimens. Multiple seizure types occurring in the affected individual, a grossly abnormal neurologic examination, or a low intelligence quotient lessen the probability that the epilepsy will be controlled with one drug or a combination of drugs [3, 6]. When a discrete event caused the seizure disorder to develop, the type of event will correlate with the probability of seizure control. Epilepsy developing secondary to massive head trauma is not likely to abate completely on any antiepileptic regimen [6]. Individuals in whom strokes or central nervous system infections coincided with the appearance of their seizure disorders usually are well controlled with a single antiepileptic drug.

Probably more important than any other factor in determining the level of seizure control achieved is the type of epilepsy exhibited by the patient. Individuals with some types of partial seizures uncomplicated by tonic-clonic convulsions have a fairly high rate of seizure control on drugs [5]. However, there are numerous reports of problems with seizure control in patients with complex partial seizures; some estimates indicate that control may be complete in only 20 to 30 percent of patients [6].

Anticipating which patients will face problems with seizure control limits the frustration and disenchantment common to individuals who expect a reprieve that fails to arrive. Electrical studies of the brain may help define the patients who will respond most poorly to antiepileptic medication. Patients with electroencephalographic abnormalities in the anterior temporal or frontal lobes have poor rates of seizure control [5]. Patients with only minor electroencephalographic abnormalities in the background on multiple recordings have good rates of seizure control.

With appropriate antiepileptic regimens, complete elimination of seizures is possible in 40 to 60 percent of individuals with partial seizures [5, 7]. Control of seizures is achieved in 69 to 75 percent of patients with generalized tonic-clonic (grand mal) epilepsy [5, 7]. This is about the same as the level of control attainable in generalized absence (petit mal) seizures [5]. Considering all seizure types together, one finds that only 9 percent or so of patients on standard antiepileptic regimens will show no response to the drugs, and at least 58 percent experience excellent seizure control (Table 12–5) [5].

The patient's general examination provides some insight into the likelihood of future seizure activity while he is on antiepileptic drugs. The less evidence there is of brain damage on clinical as well as electrical studies, the more likely it is that the patient will achieve full seizure control. The absence of intellectual or personality disorders improves the chances that epileptic activity can be completely suppressed [5].

The poorest chances of seizure control are seen in patients who have intellectual deficits associated with their seizure disorders and in patients who develop epilepsy before they are 12 months old [5]. This excludes febrile seizures, a problem common in infants and not indicative of long-term epilepsy. The poor outcome with seizures appearing before 1 year of age is probably due to the high probability of congenital brain damage in this group of patients.

An especially worrisome sign is the association of a profoundly abnormal electroencephalogram (hypsarrhythmia) with body and limb jerks (infantile spasms) in the newborn. Infants with hypsarrhythmia may develop brain

Table 12–5.
Predictors of Poor Seizure Control

History of infantile spasms
Multiple seizure types
Complex partial seizures that secondarily generalize
Signs of structural brain damage
Persistent anterior temporal or frontal EEG abnormalities
Nonfebrile seizure onset before 1 year of age
Delayed antiepileptic drug treatment

damage if treatment of seizures is delayed even a few days, but even with early treatment of these children with infantile spasms, the outlook is poor (see Chapter 13) [6].

The more closely patients are followed by physicians, the better their seizure control tends to be [5]. This is obviously a somewhat circular phenomenon, since patients willing to see a physician often are also more willing to comply with the physician's instructions than are individuals resistant to medical advice. When seizure control is poor, the patient is more likely to be skeptical of the physician's approach and more often experiments with unorthodox approaches to the problem. Despite the reluctance of those most in need of supervision to submit to it, a substantial difference in seizure control can be achieved in cases in which the physician makes a concerted effort to monitor the patient directly or through the cooperation of the patient's family.

DISCONTINUING MEDICATION

There are patients who will remain seizure-free for several years with antiepileptic drug treatment and who will remain seizure-free after the antiepileptics are discontinued. Guidelines for discontinuing medication in children with seizures were discussed in Chapter 10. Those guidelines are obviously incomplete and somewhat ambiguous, but they should become more precise as different types of epilepsy are better defined and their natural histories are better understood.

Those patients most likely to have a remission include children with rolandic epilepsy and individuals with early posttraumatic seizures [1, 8]. Those least likely ever to be independent of antiepileptic drugs include individuals with frequent seizures, persistently poor seizure control on good medication regimens, abnormal intellectual function, or repeated episodes of tonic-clonic status epilepticus [1]. If a child has rolandic or generalized absence seizures that have been completely controlled for 2 years, medication can be withdrawn. Most physicians recommend that this be attempted after only 2 years of control only if the electroencephalogram is normal [2]. The patient may remain seizure-free even if the electroencephalogram is abnormal, but a normal brain wave pattern provides an additional argument for discontinuing drugs in a patient who probably can manage without medication.

With simple partial, complex partial, and generalized tonic-clonic epilepsies, a seizure-free interval of at least 4 years should pass before medications are stopped [1]. Medications probably cannot ever be safely discontinued with benign juvenile myoclonic seizures and other generalized seizures in which tonic-clonic activity is complicated by an initial clonic phase [1].

If seizure control has been complete for 2 to 5 years, many physicians and most patients favor stopping the antiepileptic drugs. This is not without risks. The likelihood that seizure activity will recur after medication is stopped varies with the type of seizure disorder. Five to 25 percent of generalized absence seizures will recur within 5 years of drug termination [7]. If the patient had generalized tonic-clonic seizures as well as absence seizures, the risk of recurrent seizure activity off all medication is 65 percent [7]. With benign juvenile myoclonic epilepsy, the probability that the patient will remain seizure-free for 5 years after antiepileptic use is discontinued is only 5 to 25 percent, but with simple partial seizures, the likelihood is 75 percent if the seizures can be controlled for so long an interval [7]. Sixty to 80 percent of tonic-clonic seizures that typically occur while the patient is awake will return within 5 years of stopping medication, and 50 to 85 percent of complex partial seizures will recur after medication is stopped [7].

ALTERNATIVES TO DRUGS

Patients anxious for quick resolution of the epilepsy often turn to the alternatives discussed in Chapter 15. Some of these are reasonable, but many are just quackery. It is wise for the physician to discuss with the patient many of the options available, even if they will never be necessary. For the patient who is doing well on drugs, alternatives become irrelevant. For those who are doing poorly, the knowledge that there are other ways of treating the seizures, even if they are too extreme to consider until the drugs have been used for years, may limit their despair and improve their compliance.

REFERENCES

1. Delgado-Escueta, A.V., Treiman, D.M., Walsh, G. The treatable epilepsies (part 2). *N. Engl. J. Med.* 308(26):1576–1584, 1983.
2. Millichap, J.G. Drug Treatment of convulsive disorders. *N. Engl. J. Med.* 286(9): 464–469, 1972.
3. Shorvon, S.D., Reynolds, E.H. Early prognosis of epilepsy. *Br. Med. J.* 285(6356):1699–1702, 1982.
4. Goodridge, D.M.G., Shorvon, S.D. Epileptic seizures in a population of 6000. *Br. Med. J. [Clin. Res.]* 287:641–647, 1983.
5. Okuma, T., Kumashiro, H. Natural history and prognosis of epilepsy: report of a multi-institutional study in Japan. *Epilepsia* 22:35–53, 1981.
6. Rodin, E.A. *The Prognosis of Patients with Epilepsy.* Springfield, Ill. Charles C. Thomas, 1968, p. 455.
7. Delgado-Escueta, A.V., Treiman, D.M., Walsh, G.O. The treatable epilepsies (part 1). *N. Engl. J. Med.* 308(25):1508–1514, 1983.
8. Jennett, B. Epilepsy after head injury and craniotomy. In Godwin-Austen, R.B. Espir, M.L.E. (eds.), *Driving and Epilepsy.* Royal Society of Medicine International Congress and Sympasium Series, no. 60. London: Academic Press, 1983, pp. 49–51.

13. Treatment of Specific Seizure Disorders

Different types of seizure disorders demand different therapeutic approaches. The therapeutic approach to generalized tonic-clonic seizures that occur once monthly is not appropriate for the same type of seizures occurring every 5 minutes. The therapy must be dictated by the immediate and long-term risks facing the patient, as well as by the likelihood that a simple approach will be effective. Status epilepticus and neonatal seizures demand immediate and aggressive therapeutic intervention. In contrast, an isolated seizure in a young child with a high fever may demand no immediate antiepileptic treatment. For most situations in which seizures occur, there is general agreement on what constitutes essential or appropriate treatment.

NONFEBRILE SEIZURES IN INFANTS

If an infant develops seizures independent of any fever, the seizures are more likely to require energetic and long-term treatment than if they occur strictly in association with a fever. Some febrile seizures are from meningitis or encephalitis, and so no febrile seizure should be dismissed as benign, but nonfebrile seizures are even more worrisome than febrile seizures and generally warrant antiepileptic treatment.

Neonatal Seizures

Seizures in the newborn period demand immediate attention and therapy. The investigation and treatment of the neonate should progress concurrently because of the substantial risk of permanent damage if treatment is delayed at all [1, 2]. How well the infant ultimately will do is determined by the speed and appropriateness of the treatment, as well as by the etiology of the seizures (see Chapter 5). Attention must be paid to the mother's history and health, as well as to the infant's problems, because at this stage the two individuals are still affected by one another's problems. The condition of the child's mother long before the delivery may suggest that neonatal seizures will occur.

Emergency Measures
At the first sign of neonatal seizure activity, the child should undergo emergency blood studies that will check at least for serum glucose, electrolytes, urea nitrogen, and creatinine (see Table 6–1). The electrolytes examined should include calcium and magnesium. No child should be exposed to profound hypoglycemia for any longer than is absolutely necessary, but the blind administration of hypertonic glucose solutions intravenously, a practice that is routine in some institutions, has its own drawbacks. Among other complications, giving hypertonic fluids to the newborn will increase the risk of intracranial hemorrhage, a risk that is already substantial in premature infants. Rapid determination of serum glucose usually is practical with colorimetric strip testing (Dextrostix). If serum glucose appears to be normal or high, the child can be spared the risks of a glucose infusion. If it is low, a 25% glucose solution can be administered (Table 13–1).

If an emergency lumbar puncture suggests meningitis, intravenous antibiotic therapy should be started immediately, with primary therapy directed against group B beta-hemolytic streptococci if the neonate is full-term and against gram-negative organisms if the infant is premature [1]. If the cerebrospinal fluid is bloody, computed tomography may help establish the source of the bleeding.

Some physicians recommend using calcium gluconate and magnesium sulfate injections for all children with neonatal seizures, but this may be unnecessary if laboratory studies can be completed within minutes of the child's initial seizure. The physician without emergency laboratory facilities may be obliged to provide these electrolytes and subsequently determine whether they were necessary. If the child has hyponatremia, inappropriate antidiuretic hormone associated with a meningitis usually is responsible, and the finding of a normal cerebrospinal fluid should be questioned. If the patient is dehydrated and has hypernatremia, rehydration should be begun immediately [1].

The best way to check for pyridoxine dependence is to monitor seizure activity while pyridoxine is infused [1]. Screening tests of serum amino acid

Table 13–1.
Management of Neonatal Seizures

Emergency serum glucose measurement
Solution of 25% dextrose in water I.V. at 0.5 to 1.0 g/kg if hypoglycemic
Emergency calcium determination
5% calcium gluconate I.V. at 200 mg/kg if hypocalcemic
50% magnesium sulfate I.M. at 0.2 ml/kg if hypomagnesemic
Trial of pyridoxine 50 mg I.V. with electroencephalographic monitor
Emergency lumbar puncture

If seizures persist
Loading dose of phenobarbital I.V. 15 mg/kg
Additional phenobarbital I.V. 5 mg/kg up to a maximum of 40 mg/kg
Loading dose of phenytoin I.V. 10 mg/kg
Additional dose of phenytoin I.V. up to a maximum of 20 mg/kg

If needed
Maintenance dextrose I.V. at up to 0.5 g/kg/hr
Maintenance phenobarbital I.V. 2.5 mg/kg every 12 hours
Maintenance phenytoin I.V. 2.5 mg/kg every 12 hours
Maintenance pyridoxine I.V. 10 mg/kg/day
Intravenous antibiotics to treat meningoencephalitis

Routinely
Monitor serum antiepileptic drug levels
Maintain serum phenobarbital level at 20–30 μg/ml for 2 weeks or until the neonate is stable
Support blood pressure and respiration at all times
Stop antiepileptics after seizures stop only if no neurologic deficits or developmental delays
  are found

I.V. = intravenously; I.M. = intramuscularly.

levels may point to an inborn error of metabolism Serum phenylalanine levels usually will be high enough at the time of the initial seizure to allow phenylketonuria to be diagnosed. Dietary precautions to minimize the level of phenylalanine in the diet should be instituted as soon as phenylketonuria is recognized as a problem. Most other genetically determined metabolic problems, such as maple syrup urine disease, are not treatable, but management of the child with such untreatable conditions may be simplified by administering phenobarbital as an antiepileptic if the child can tolerate it. Throughout the management of the seizures, the child's blood pressure and ventilation should be monitored and maintained [1].

Antiepileptic Drugs
If there is no readily reversible cause for the seizures, the child should be given antiepileptic medication immediately [3]. Phenobarbital is the drug of choice and should be given intravenously if that is practical [2]. Intrarectal or intramuscular phenobarbital is well absorbed during the neonatal period and may provide substantial anticonvulsant protection until an intravenous route is established. In fact, phenobarbital's major advantage over other medications is that it is quickly absorbed regardless of the route of administration and rapidly exerts its effect in the neonatal brain [2].

A loading dose of 15 mg/kg is followed every 5 to 10 minutes by an additional dose of 5 to 10 mg/kg up to a maximum of 40 mg/kg or until the seizures stop [3]. Phenobarbital alone should be used unless the seizures are not controlled even when the serum phenobarbital level reaches 40 μg/ml. Seizures controlled with phenobarbital alone usually will remain well controlled with serum phenobarbital levels at 20 to 30 μg/ml.

If phenobarbital does not stop the seizures, phenytoin at no more than 3 mg/kg/min should be added. The phenytoin infusion rate that very small children can tolerate is not as great or as consistent as that tolerated by adults, and so cardiac activity must be closely monitored while the drug is slowly infused. An initial dose of 50 to 100 mg of phenytoin may suffice to stop the seizures. Phenytoin is effective only if it is given intravenously, and some infants tolerate it poorly regardless of the precautions taken [2]. Other drugs used in these children include diazepam, introduced as an intrarectal solution at 0.25 to 0.50 mg/kg, and paraldehyde as a 2% solution at 0.2 ml/kg [2].

Phenobarbital does stop neonatal seizures in 85 percent of cases. The group of newborns who respond most poorly to this drug alone are those who suffered prolonged asphyxia before or at the time of birth [3]. Unfortunately, hypoxic or ischemic brain disease causes more neonatal seizures than any other single problem.

Many causes of neonatal seizures have fairly transient effects. Even asphyxia need not cause persistent seizures. In most cases, phenobarbital is not needed for more than 2 weeks, but some physicians recommend continuing its use for 3 months [2]. After the drug is stopped, the seizures generally do not recur [3].

Side effects of phenobarbital given to the newborn include depressed activity and muscle tone, but it is often difficult to determine whether the hypotonia and hypoactivity are due to the drug or to the central nervous system lesion [3]. The use of any antiepileptic medication during the newborn period is complicated by the infant's unusual handling of drugs. Unlike older children and adults with epilepsy, the neonate with seizures does not seem to establish a steady state or stable level of antiepileptic in the blood [4]. Half-lives of drugs like phenytoin range from 4 to 140 hours when measured directly [4]. This means that routine expectations about what will be an adequate loading dose and what is an appropriate maintenance dose cannot be applied when the patient is a newborn. Frequent measurements of serum antiepileptic levels are a substantial aid in managing these infants.

Infantile Spasms

Although infantile spasms are actually a collection of different seizure types, the infants with this syndrome of generalized seizures associated with paroxysms of muscle activity and diffusely abnormal encephalographic records are all best treated with adrenocorticotropic hormone (ACTH) [5]. The reasons for the effectiveness of ACTH in managing these seizures are unknown, but that it is effective with at least some patients is well established [5, 6]. Adrenocorticotropic hormone affects the pace and pattern of maturation in the brain and probably exerts its influence at this level [6]. It has not worked as an antiepileptic in adults or older children (see Chapter 14).

Infants with infantile spasms who are treated early with high doses of ACTH have less psychomotor retardation and a lower incidence of later epilepsy than children not treated early or at all [5]. There is no evidence that a delay of hours in the initiation of treatment causes any damage to the child, and so the start of therapy can and should follow a careful evaluation of the infant to ascertain that treatment is appropriate. Before ACTH therapy is instituted, the child must be evaluated for central nervous system and systemic infections, since the immunosuppressant effect of the drug could be life-threatening if the child already has an infection [5].

Ideally, the hormone should be started within 1 or 2 days of the onset of the seizures, with an initial dose of 110 units/m^2/day of the ACTH gel given intramuscularly or an equivalent dose of the solution given intravenously [5]. This dose is continued for 3 weeks before it is tapered to 70 units/m^2/day. After 2 weeks of this dose, the ACTH is again reduced to 50 units/m^2/day administered every other day for 3 more weeks [5].

Valproate sodium (valproic acid), phenobarbital, or benzodiazepines often are given in conjunction with the ACTH if infantile spasms persist despite the hormone treatment [6]. That these additional antiepileptics substantially affect the long-term outcome is unlikely [5], but they do suppress much of the seizure activity that increases the child's risk of injury or aspiration.

The longterm effects of ACTH are unknown, but until a better treatment is found, it will remain the first-line drug [6]. Severe side effects develop over the short term in approximately 37 percent of the infants given ACTH [6]. Most of these reflect high levels of steroid production induced by the hormone. Hirsutism, sleep disturbances, moon facies, and hypertension are especially common problems. Regardless of how these infants are treated, many die, and of those that survive, 80 to 90 percent are mentally retarded [6].

FEBRILE SEIZURES

In infants with simple febrile seizures, the treatment of choice is fever reduction. This can usually be achieved with antipyretic medication, such as aspirin, and topical coolants, such as alcohol rubs and water baths. Children with complex febrile seizures should be investigated to determine the basis for the seizures, and if the cause is not completely reversible, the child should be given antiepileptic drugs. Most physicians consider phenobarbital the drug of choice for managing complex febrile seizures [7].

In the past, many physicians tried to suppress simple febrile seizures in a child with a history of one or more of these episodes by giving the child phenobarbital whenever a fever developed. This is no longer the accepted treatment for simple febrile seizures, because anticonvulsant levels are achieved too slowly to make a difference when the child is acutely sick unless the drugs are given intravenously or intramuscularly each time a fever appears. The complication rate for intravenous antiepileptic treatment is too high to justify its use in prophylaxis of simple febrile seizures. Some physicians do use intermittent diazepam or clonazepam to manage simple febrile seizures that appear repeatedly, but most prefer to avoid anticonvulsant medications altogether [8].

With complex febrile seizures, the child usually is maintained on therapeutic doses of phenobarbital for several years. This approach will prevent febrile seizures in 80 percent of the children treated, but most of these children will also exhibit adverse reactions to the drug [8]. The commonest reactions are irritability, hyperactivity, negativistic behavior, sleep disturbances, and rashes. At least 13 percent of the children treated with fairly low doses of phenobarbital will tolerate the drug so poorly that the dosage must be dropped.

Because of the side effects of phenobarbital, children with complex febrile seizures have been tried on a variety of other drugs. Trials using primidone have shown this drug to be more effective than phenobarbital in suppressing seizure activity, and the incidence of adverse reactions is much lower [8]. The adverse reactions that occur with primidone are the same as those occurring with phenobarbital, a finding that is not surprising, since primidone is partly metabolized to phenobarbital. Carbamazepine and phenytoin are not at all useful in the management of febrile convulsions.

Valproic acid (valproate sodium) is effective in suppressing complex febrile seizures in more than 91 percent of cases and produces noticeable side effects in only 45 percent of children [8]. These reactions include nausea, vomiting, anorexia, irritability, and polyuria. Despite the obvious advantages of valproic acid from the standpoint of efficacy, many physicians are uncomfortable with reports of liver or pancreatic disease in isolated cases [8]. The risk to the child probably is not substantial, but in any child given this drug, liver and pancreatic enzymes should be monitored.

Regardless of which drug is used, as many as 1 in 5 parents will stop the anticonvulsants without consulting their child's physician [9]. This failure to comply with a physician's instructions probably reflects the parents' concerns about giving an infant medication when he is not having seizures.

WEST AND LENNOX-GASTAUT SYNDROMES

How best to treat West syndrome and the closely related disorder of Lennox-Gastaut syndrome is controversial, but there is a consensus that none of the presently available therapies is very useful. Because these are symptomatic epilepsies, the best approach is prevention, but this is not practical. Even if intrauterine infections, perinatal hypoxia, subarachnoid hemorrhage, and perinatal trauma could be eliminated, children would still develop these syndromes for no apparent reason or as a consequence of congenital malformations. Drugs are needed to suppress the seizures evident in the children with either of these syndromes, and none of the currently available agents seems to improve the prognosis substantially.

Adrenocorticotropic hormone is the drug of choice for the infantile spasms characteristically seen in West syndrome, but, as already mentioned, the high doses of this hormone required to suppress the seizures may produce signs of hyperadrenocorticism. Still, ACTH provides the best hope for suppressing infantile spasms, and it does seem to improve the prognosis slightly.

Less effective but less hazardous drugs that will produce symptomatic improvement in many of the children with West syndrome include valproic acid and clonazepam [10]. The long-term effects of these drugs on infants remain to be established.

Children who develop the Lennox-Gastaut syndrome are usually older than those with West syndrome. Phenobarbital often is preferred for management of the seizures in these children, but valproic acid or phenytoin are reasonable alternatives. As the child matures and other types of seizures appear, the antiepileptic regimen should be changed to include the most effective drug for the seizure type that the patient exhibits most often.

BENIGN JUVENILE MYOCLONIC EPILEPSY

Benign juvenile myoclonic epilepsy usually is fairly sensitive to medication. The drug of choice for this type of seizure is valproic acid, but if this drug cannot be tolerated, clonazepam is usually safe and effective. Patients with associated absence seizures may need treatment with ethosuximide, and patients not well controlled on any of these drugs alone may profit from drug combinations including phenytoin [11].

Although these seizures usually abate as the adolescent matures, they do not remit completely. Most patients remain well controlled while on antiepileptic medication [11]. Long-term antiepileptic treatment appears to be unavoidable, but whether drugs should be continued for more than 4 years after the last seizure occurs has not been determined. Most patients stop taking the medications regardless of what they are advised to do, and the typical consequence is that the seizures reappear within a few months or years.

ROLANDIC EPILEPSY

Benign focal epilepsy of childhood, or rolandic epilepsy, usually is easily suppressed with one antiepileptic drug, but sometimes this type of epilepsy need not be treated at all. In most of the affected children, seizure activity is limited almost exclusively to when they are asleep. The seizures disappear by the end of adolescence whether or not the patient is treated, and none of the antiepileptics used for these partial seizures is without its own risks.

Most physicians will treat these seizures with valproic acid or phenytoin if the child has more than two or three seizures while he is awake. After no seizures have occurred for 2 or 3 years, the antiepileptic may be tapered. If seizures are going to recur, they will usually begin as nocturnal seizures. These pose little risk to the child but can be used as an indicator that antiepileptic medication should not yet be discontinued.

MANAGEMENT OF AN EPILEPTIC EPISODE

When a seizure occurs, the primary physician, whether a neurologist, pediatrician, family practitioner, internist, or other type of doctor, is routinely asked about management. The concerned family may expect the patient to be hospitalized. Doctors and nurses who are unfamiliar with epilepsy and who witness an episode in the hospital may initiate resuscitation with intubation of the convulsing patient. The appropriate measures for immediate seizure management depend primarily on the type of seizure and its context.

If the patient is having a generalized absence seizure and the same type of seizure has occurred 10 times in 2 days, all the physician need do is manipulate the patient's medication in an attempt to achieve better seizure control. If the patient has never had a seizure before and a generalized tonic-clonic seizure occurs, that patient should be hospitalized for investigation and observation. Even if the patient has a long history of tonic-clonic seizures with past episodes of status epilepticus, every episode of status epilepticus justifies emergency admission to a hospital and the institution of drug therapy on the way to the emergency facility.

The most frightening seizure episode is the generalized tonic-clonic seizure or convulsion. It usually starts with little warning, and the patient may injure himself during the inevitable fall to the ground. Generally, by the time the convulsion is recognized for what it is, the patient's jaws are locked shut. It is commonly believed that something should be forced into the mouth to separate the teeth and protect the tongue, but attempts to do this after the patient's mouth is firmly closed result in teeth being knocked out and aspirated. It is usually best not to force anything into the mouth if it cannot be placed between the teeth without a struggle.

The patient's forceful clonic movements should not be suppressed, and any tonic posturing should not be resisted. It is often useful to get the patient onto his side to minimize aspiration of food or secretions, but this should not be done if it requires a struggle with the patient. Shoulder dislocations also occur in some generalized convulsions, and so any manipulation of the patient should not involve pulling on his arm.

Even if the fall does not injure the patient, the force of his own tonic-clonic muscle contractions may fracture susceptible bones. Old women with severe osteoporosis are at high risk for compression fractures of the vertebrae. The thrashing limb and trunk movements can produce additional injury if solid objects are in the way. Dangerous objects should be moved away or, if that is not possible, the patient should be moved away from the objects. Cushioning the patient's head and other body surfaces as much as possible will reduce injuries, but this usually is not practical. In any case, the patient's head should be kept from banging against the ground during the convulsion.

If the patient has an aura that allows seizures to be recognized before the ictus is entered, additional precautions may be taken. The patient should be placed on the ground or on a flat uncluttered surface before the seizure generalizes. Confused patients may resist this until it is too late, but many will cooperate. If the disorder involves seizures that secondarily generalize, a well-padded object, such as a tongue depressor wrapped in gauze, should be placed in the mouth to interfere with tongue biting. If a physician or nurse is at hand he or she may insert a plastic airway instead, which is preferable because it will keep the tongue from falling back or being inadvertently forced back into the throat.

With any generalized seizure, the patient usually becomes cyanotic, and breathing appears to be labored. These disturbing signs pass within a minute or two, and the patient does not need to be intubated. Intubation will be difficult during this stage anyway, because the jaw will be closed tightly and the patient will be posturing or thrashing about. By the time intubation becomes practical, it usually is obvious that the patient is not having respiratory difficulty.

After the generalized convulsion, most patients are very confused. The recovering patient should be surrounded by as little tumult as possible and encouraged to stay where he is until confusion has cleared completely. Restraining the patient usually is self-defeating, since it only serves to agitate the confused individual and he may inadvertently injure himself or the people trying to restrain him.

He should not be given anything to drink or eat until the postictal confusion has abated considerably. Premature efforts to get the patient to drink some stimulant leads to aspiration. There is no beverage, alcoholic or otherwise, that will speed the patient's rate of recovery. Many patients feel exhausted after a generalized convulsion. Their desire to sleep should not be frustrated, but they should be watched for recurrent seizure activity.

If this is one of many seizures, it is a signal that the patient's medication must be adjusted or his compliance checked. This generally does not require hospitalization. However, if seizures are occurring several times per week, hospitalization may be needed so that abrupt changes in medication dosages may be made and supervised. Hospitalization provides an opportunity not only for monitoring adverse reactions to changes in a patient's drug regimen but also for investigating the basis for the increasing seizure frequency. As previously mentioned, when the patient has the first seizure of his life, it is prudent to hospitalize him and watch for meningitis or other rapidly progressive neurologic problems.

ANTIEPILEPTIC THERAPY WITH SUBSTANCE ABUSE

Seizures associated with alcohol or drug abuse have been a common problem in many countries, including the United States, for decades. Recently, though, there have been changes in the spectrum of drugs commonly involved. Alcohol has been the substance most frequently involved in addiction-related seizures for more than a century, and it continues to lead all other drugs in frequency of its abuse. Some of the illicit agents in current use, such as marijuana, are not associated with an increased risk of seizures, but others, such as barbiturates and cocaine, carry substantial risks.

If an abuser of alcohol, barbiturates, amphetamines, cocaine, or other drugs has a seizure for the first time in his life, the cause of that seizure must be investigated as vigorously as any seizure unrelated to substance abuse. That the patient was exposed to an agent which could lower his seizure threshold while he was taking it or when he stopped using it does not eliminate the possibility that a brain tumor, vascular malformation, central nervous system infection, or other central nervous system disorder contributed to the seizure disorder. The investigation of the patient with a history of substance abuse is complicated, because the effects of intoxication with, or withdrawal from, the substance must be managed at the same time that the seizure disorder is investigated.

Whenever alcohol abuse is suspected in a patient who has been hospitalized, thiamine hydrochloride, 100 mg intramuscularly, should be given prophylactically for 4 days to minimize the risk of damage from Wernicke's encephalopathy, an often disabling and occasionally lethal central nervous system disorder [12]. Although the thiamine will reduce the risk of neurologic deficits, such as memory impairment, ocular motor abnormalities, and gait difficulty, it will not eliminate the risk of seizures as the serum alcohol level falls. Patients who are still clearly intoxicated also may develop alcohol-related seizures, and so a high blood alcohol level should not be taken as a sign that there is time to manage the patient before he is likely to have a seizure.

Patients who have been alcoholics for years should routinely be given drugs to suppress the withdrawal syndrome associated with interrupted alcohol abuse. Many physicians use chlordiazepoxide as the initial drug to minimize the risk of delirium tremens, but phenobarbital, 100 to 200 mg intramuscularly, is equally effective and has the added advantage of suppressing seizures during alcohol withdrawal.

With other types of substance abuse that may cause seizures, the initial management of the patient must focus on stabilizing the vital signs while minimizing the risk of seizures. If barbiturates have been abused, the individual should be given 200 mg phenobarbital intramuscularly, with gradual withdrawal of this supplementary barbiturate. If signs of withdrawal, such as twitching, tremors, or agitation, are already obvious at the time the patient is initially examined, a 300-mg dose of phenobarbital may be needed to minimize the risk of seizures [13].

If the patient has taken an overdose of methaqualone (Quaalude), he may have seizures, but autonomic instability presents as great a threat to the patient. Blood pressure, body temperature, ventilation, and cardiac activity must all be monitored [13]. If a seizure occurs, the patient should be given intramuscular phenobarbital at an initial dose of 100 mg, but prophylactic barbiturates are not appropriate.

Autonomic problems are even more of a threat with amphetamine or cocaine abuse. If seizures develop while the patient is using these agents, the patients should be given intramuscular phenobarbital. Because amphetamines and cocaine often are sold as highly adulterated preparations, the patient should be observed for other toxic effects of the abused substance.

MANAGING STATUS EPILEPTICUS

Status epilepticus can be lethal if it is not treated, but with appropriate management, the patient usually will recover. The basic feature of status epilepticus is that the seizure activity occurs repeatedly without adequately protracted intervals between seizures to allow the patient to recover fully normal functioning. If the patient has idiopathic epilepsy, the probable cause of the status epilepticus is poor drug compliance. If status epilepticus is the first sign of a seizure disorder, then an explanation for the seizures must be sought rapidly.

Treatment of status epilepticus demands intravenous antiepileptic drugs at high doses. There are many different methods for managing this problem, and several are equally effective. The most important element in any treatment plan is speed. The cause of the seizures must be quickly assessed and appropriate treatment begun. If no history is available on the patient, the investigation of the patient may be more protracted, but treatment should not be delayed even when the etiology of the status epilepticus is uncertain.

Tonic-Clonic Status Epilepticus

As soon as status epilepticus is recognized, the patient must be stabilized. This means placing an airway, maintaining an effective blood pressure, checking for cardiac arrhythmias, starting treatment for hyperthermia or hypothermia, and checking arterial blood gases [14]. If any autonomic function is grossly abnormal, attempts should be made to correct it at the same time that the

Table 13–2.
Treatment Guidelines in Status Epilepticus

Stabilize autonomic functions
Check blood gases and chemistries
Start intravenous drug therapy
Intubate if breathing appears compromised or if arterial blood gases are poor
Monitor vital signs
Proceed with diagnostic studies as quickly as feasible

seizures are being treated Table 13–2. Some physicians recommend giving an intravenous bolus of 50% glucose solution (50ml) and an intramuscular injection of thiamine (100mg) [14]. These two measures will help protect the patient from hypoglycemia or Wernicke's encephalopathy, problems that may not be evident until after substantial brain damage has occurred.

If the patient has been on antiepileptic drugs prior to the development of status epilepticus, some of the blood drawn to check the patient's electrolyte, glucose, calcium, hemoglobin, and hematocrit levels, and white blood cell count should be assessed also for anticonvulsant drug levels. This will be important later when the physician and patient are trying to determine what caused the episode of status epilepticus.

In most cases, a combination of phenytoin and diazepam is enough to stop the recurrent seizure activity. Initially, 500 mg phenytoin is delivered intravenously at a rate not greater than 50 mg/min in the adult. If seizure activity does not abate with this dose, 10 mg diazepam intravenously should be given and repeated every 10 minutes up to a total dose of 50 mg. Many neurologists prefer to administer an intravenous dose of diazepam first, but it is always wise to give the patient phenytoin as well, because the diazepam is cleared too quickly from the blood to provide long-term protection against recurrent seizures (Table 13–3) [14].

The patient's breathing, blood pressure, and electrocardiogram must be monitored throughout this treatment. If there is any evidence that breathing is being depressed by the medications, the patient should be intubated and placed on a ventilator. If seizures persist, another 500 mg phenytoin at 50

Table 13–3.
Drug Treatment of Status Epilepticus

Glucose (50% dextrose in water) 50 ml I.V. unless history dictates against this
Thiamine 100 mg I.M. unless history dictates against this
Phenytoin 20 mg/kg I.V. at no more than 50 mg/min
Diazepam 10 mg I.V. at 2 mg/min; repeated with recurrent seizures up to a maximum of 50 mg for 1 day
Phenobarbital 260 mg I.V. at 100 mg/min; if seizures persist, repeat up to 20 mg/kg over 1 hour
Paraldehyde I.V. drip of 2 or 4% solution in normal saline; titrate to suppress seizure activity

I.V. = intravenously; I.M. = intramuscularly.

mg/min may be needed. If this fails, a 2 or 4% solution of paraldehyde in normal saline may be infused at a rate sufficient to stop the seizures. Disadvantages of paraldehyde are that it requires special tubing and must be protected from light.

Some physicians use phenobarbital in doses of 350 mg intravenously up to a maximum of 1 g over 45 minutes as an alternative to phenytoin or in addition to phenytoin and diazepam. With this much medication, the patient often will require intubation. Phenobarbital has the advantage of being more easily administered than paraldehyde. If all these measures have failed to suppress the seizure activity, it is likely that a progressive lesion in the brain is causing the status epilepticus, and no treatment short of general anesthesia will stop the seizures. Even with general anesthesia, the systemic signs of seizure activity may be suppressed while the electrical abnormality in the brain may persist unabated.

Alternative drugs include lidocaine hydrochloride and lorazepam. Fifty to 100 mg lidocaine in 250 ml of 5% dextrose in water may be delivered at 2 mg/min without much risk of cardiac toxicity, but that it truly suppresses seizure activity is uncertain [14]. Its principal action may be as a general anesthetic. Lorazepam at a dose of 0.1 mg/kg as a single intravenous injection may stop tonic-clonic status epilepticus without the use of other medications. Some physicians use lorazepam rather than diazepam or phenytoin as the initial drug.

Any patient with refractory status epilepticus should be reevaluated for metabolic or infectious bases for the seizures. Persistent hypocalcemia will interfere with seizure control more than a subarachnoid hemorrhage. The patient in whom an initial lumbar puncture is normal may have evidence of meningitis when the lumbar puncture is repeated after 12 hours. Persistent status epilepticus requires persistent efforts to identify the basis for the seizures.

Nonconvulsive Status Epilepticus

The relatively rare nonconvulsive status epilepticus syndromes are also treated with intravenous medication, but the dramatic measures needed to stabilize the patient with tonic-clonic status epilepticus generally are not necessary. Petit mal status epilepticus can usually be managed with intravenous diazepam followed by oral ethosuximide, valproic acid, or both. Complex partial status epilepticus may respond to intravenous phenytoin or diazepam.

These conditions should be treated with antiepileptic medication just as vigorously as tonic-clonic status epilepticus, but because the seizures are not convulsive, it is more difficult to be sure when the patient has been adequately treated. However, these nonconvulsive forms of status epilepticus are not likely to be lethal if they are treated only partially, and so the physician has more time to adjust the patient's medication and check for his response to treatment. Continuous electroencephalographic recording with concurrent video monitoring is especially useful in managing these nonconvulsive forms, because both the patient's long-term electroencephalographic record and minor clinical signs of continued seizure activity can be observed and correlated.

Epilepsia partialis continua—that is, simple partial status epilepticus—usually produces much less dramatic changes in the patient's clinical appearance than the other forms of status epilepticus, but it often is much more refractory to treatment. Persistent twitching in an arm or leg caused by simple partial motor status epilepticus may persist for weeks or months despite intravenous and oral medications. Several different treatment regimens have been tried with this problem, but none has produced consistently good results. The best that can be done for the patient is a systematic trial of different antiepileptic medications until one is found that suppresses the seizure activity.

REFERENCES

1. Volpe, J. J. Neonatal seizures. *Clin. Perinatol.* 4(1):43–63, 1977.
2. Aicardi, J. Neonatal and infantile seizures. In Morselli, P.L., Pippenger, C.E., Penry, J.K. (eds.), *Antiepileptic Drug Therapy in Pediatrics.* New York: Raven Press, 1983, pp. 103–113.
3. Gal, P., Toback, J., Boer, H.R., et al. Efficacy of phenobarbital monotherapy in treatment of neonatal seizures—relationship to blood levels. *Neurology* (N.Y.) 32(12):1401–1404, 1982.
4. Dodson, W.E., Bourgeois, B.F.D., Ferrendelli, J.A. Phenobarbital and phenytoin in neonatal seizures. *Neurology* (N.Y.) 32(12):1405, 1982.
5. Lombroso, C.T. A prospective study of infantile spasms: clinical and therapeutic correlations. *Epilepsia* 24(2):135–158, 1983.
6. Riikonen, R. Infantile spasms: some new theoretical aspects. *Epilepsia* 24(2):159–168, 1983.
7. Drugs for epilepsy. *Med. Lett. Drugs Ther.* 25(643):81–84, 1983.
8. Herranz, J.L., Armijo, J.A., Arteaga, R. Effectiveness and toxicity of phenobarbital, primidone, and sodium valproate in the prevention of febrile convulsions, controlled by plasma levels. *Epilepsia* 25(1):89–95, 1984.
9. Febrile convulsions. *Br. Med. J.* 282(6265):673–674, 1981.
10. Delgado-Escueta, A.V., Treiman, D.M., Walsh, G.O. The treatable epilepsies (part 1). *N. Engl. J. Med.* 308(25):1508–1514, 1983.
11. Asconape, J., Penry, J.K. Some clinical and EEG aspects of benign juvenile myoclonic epilepsy. *Epilepsia* 25(1):108–114, 1984.
12. Adams, R., Victor, M. *Principles of Neurology, ed. 2.* New York: McGraw-Hill, 1981.
13. Drugs of choice. New Rochelle, N.Y.: The Medical Letter, 1977, pp. 45–63.
14. Engel, J., Jr., Troupin, A.S., Crandall, P.H., et al. Recent development in the diagnosis and therapy of epilepsy. *Ann. Intern. Med.* 97:584–598, 1982.

14. Antiepileptic Drugs

Phenobarbital was introduced in 1912 and provided dramatic relief from seizures for many patients. Its inability to suppress all seizure types and its obvious side effects, such as sedation in adults and hyperactivity in children, prompted the development of other antiepileptic agents. Combinations of several bromide salts were also found to be effective anticonvulsants, but these, too, caused sedation and had the added disadvantage of causing severe acne. Despite their disadvantages, bromides were alleged to control seizures in 78 percent of the patients treated [1]. Consistently underreported in all experiences with antiepileptic drugs is the duration of the complete control. At least partly because control was a transient phenomenon and partly because the side effects of both phenobarbital and bromides were marginally tolerable for many patients, other drugs were sought.

Phenytoin entered clinical neurology in 1938 and immediately became the standard by which all future antiepileptic drugs would be measured [2]. Most of the antiepileptics subsequently developed have had chemical ties to either phenobarbital or phenytoin (Fig. 14–1). Primidone and phenobarbital are so closely related that when primidone was first introduced, there was controversy over whether its only active metabolite was phenobarbital. Ethosuximide and methsuximide had no advantages over phenytoin in most seizure disorders, but they proved more effective than other drugs in suppressing generalized absence (petit mal) seizures. Valproic acid (valproate sodium) is one of the few antiepileptics bearing no structural similarity to phenobarbital or phenytoin.

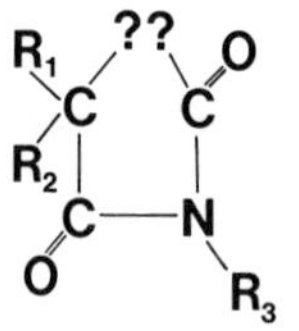

Figure 14–1.
Most antiepileptic drugs share these basic elements. R_1, R_2, and R_3 are carbon atom or phenyl group side chains. Whether the central ring will have five members or six is determined by the substitutions at ??.

It has proved valuable in treating generalized seizure disorders, but the importance of its hepatic and pancreatic toxicity remains to be determined.

All of the currently used antiepileptic drugs have numerous side effects. Most of the risks associated with the antiepileptics are the same for all individuals taking the medication, but there are some special cases. Women trying to become pregnant while taking antiepileptics must face the risk of birth defects developing in the fetus. Men with waning sexual potency may find certain drugs, such as phenobarbital, primidone, or phenytoin, eliminate the little potency they retained.

Most antiepileptics are metabolized primarily in the liver and circulate as both bound and unbound fractions in the bloodstream. Both of these facts influence how effective the drug can be and how well the patient given the drug will tolerate it in the face of nonneurologic disease. Any individual with chronic liver disease or alcoholism may be unable to tolerate drugs metabolized in the liver. Individuals requiring more than one antiepileptic in combination will face an increased risk of side effects from the individual drugs and their interactions.

PHENYTOIN

Phenytoin sodium (Dilantin, Epanutin) is an effective antiepileptic for several different generalized and partial epilepsies and is the drug of choice for generalized tonic-clonic (grand mal) epilepsy (Fig. 14–2) [3]. It is used as an alternative (second choice) drug in many types of epilepsy if more appropriate antiepileptics fail to produce good control (see Table 12–2). Most physicians use it as the initial drug in the management of status epilepticus.

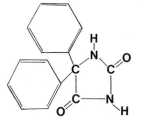

Figure 14–2.
Chemical structure of phenytoin.

Phenytoin is available as a capsule, tablet, or syrup for oral use and in solution for intravenous use. It crystallizes when it is injected into muscle, and absorption by that route is too unpredictable to be useful. It is given to both adults and children with generalized tonic-clonic seizures and is also helpful in the management of simple and complex partial seizures resistant to other medication [3].

This is a fairly inexpensive drug, because it is manufactured by many different companies, but the absorption of preparations made by different manufacturers may vary greatly. The amount that actually gets into the patient's blood must be checked with regular determination of serum phenytoin levels. This may mean twice monthly assessments during the first few months of treatment, but even after the patient has reached a stable therapeutic level, the serum level should be determined every 4 to 6 months to be sure that absorption and metabolism of the drug have not changed.

Oral phenytoin can be taken as a single dose each day, but, when it is taken this infrequently, the more slowly absorbed extended phenytoin sodium capsules (Dilantin Kapseals) are more reliable than other phenytoin capsules [3]. A therapeutic level of 10 to 20 µg/ml usually is achieved when an adult is taking 300 to 400 mg (three to four capsules) of phenytoin daily (Table 14–1) [4]. Children usually require 4 to 7 mg/kg/day of the drug, but absorption and metabolism of phenytoin is more unpredictable in children than in adults [3, 5]. The serum phenytoin level, rather than the oral dose, should be watched, especially if the patient is very young or he is taking other medications along with the phenytoin. At least in adults, the serum level should reach a plateau after the patient has been on the drug for approximately 5 days [3].

With phenytoin, as with all antiepileptic drugs, it is important to remember that therapeutic doses and reasonable rates of administration must be tailored to the patient. The adult with epilepsy usually can tolerate a phenytoin intravenous infusion rate of 50 mg/min, but this is much too fast for the infant or small child. The infusion rate with these young patients should never exceed 3 mg/kg/min and should be slower if circumstances allow (see Chapter 13).

Table 14–1.
Standard Adult Dosages for Common Antiepileptic Drugs

Drug	Dosage (mg/kg body weight/day)	Days to Steady State
Phenytoin	4–10	5–10
Carbamazepine	10–25	3–6
Valproic acid	10–70	2–4
Ethosuximide	20–40	6–12
Primidone	10–25	1–5
Phenobarbital	1–5	16–21
Clonazepam	0.03–0.1	—

The half-life and time required to achieve a steady state, if one is ever achieved, in the newborn are very different from those observed in the adult. The serum drug level must be measured directly in newborns, without reliance on predicted levels.

Epileptic patients with liver or kidney disease also pose special problems for the physician managing the epilepsy. Liver disease may impair the catabolism of phenytoin, which is para-hydroxylated in the liver, and consequently increase the serum level and the risk of toxic reactions at low oral doses. With a normal liver, the patient may develop unexpected drug toxicities, or the levels of drugs given along with the phenytoin that are also metabolized in the liver may be inadequate. The enzyme-inducing action of phenytoin is not specific for enzymes that handle only phenytoin, and so other drugs, such as warfarin sodium, may be catabolized at an unanticipated rate if the patient is already taking the antiepileptic when the additional drugs are started.

Renal diseases reduce the amount of phenytoin that is bound to protein, thereby increasing the free, and presumably active, fraction of the drug [6]. Transient renal problems, such as acute tubular necrosis that remits, may produce transient distortions in the fraction of unbound phenytoin in the serum, whereas irreversible renal failure will make the patient persistently sensitive to low doses of phenytoin [6]. With the lower serum albumin that usually develops with renal failure, phenytoin is less bound, and the amount of free drug may be high even when the serum level appears to be low. Clinical signs of toxicity may be much more helpful than the serum phenytoin levels in monitoring patients with kidney disease. If the patient receives a renal transplant that functions well, the percent of bound phenytoin will return to normal within 1 or 2 weeks of the procedure [6].

Adverse Reactions

With higher phenytoin levels, toxic signs and even increased seizure frequency may appear. Toxic effects aside from an acute allergic or gastrointestinal reaction should not arise for several hours after oral administration of the drug, because absorption is so slow that peak serum levels are not reached for approximately 4 to 8 hours after an oral dose [4]. Some patients complain that phenytoin gives them an upset stomach or altered bowel patterns, but these gastrointestinal problems usually are mild and transient. Suicide attempts with this drug are not usually successful, because gastric irritation will trigger vomiting of a massive oral dose. Most patients find it difficult to take more than 500 mg (five capsules) at one time.

Although phenytoin occasionally produces blood disorders and allergic reactions, the more commonly encountered adverse reactions are neurologic and psychiatric. A staggering gait, slurred speech, blurred vision, and mild sedation are the commonest complaints. On examination, the patient will have difficulty walking, abnormal eye movements (nystagmus), and mildly slurred speech as the serum level of the drug enters the toxic range. Years of phenytoin use often cause persistent, but mild, gait problems and sensory loss. These result from injury to peripheral nerves and the cerebellum [4, 7, 8]. Some patients will develop rash, fever, hepatitis, or lymphadenopathy from the drug [8]. Individuals with organic brain disease generally exhibit a lower tolerance for phenytoin.

Another common complaint is that the drug has cosmetic effects. Women in particular notice coarsening of facial features and darkening of limb and facial hair. Both men and women suffer with gingival hyperplasia, an overgrowth of the gums that is unslightly and leads to tooth loss (see Fig. 7–1). Acne may develop in patients of any age who are on fairly low doses of the drug [8]. When the drug is stopped, the acne and gingival hyperplasia may abate, but the hair changes usually persist.

The most worrisome adverse reactions to phenytoin are hematologic and immunologic. These are not dose-related and are no more likely if the patient has been on the drug for only a few months or as long as a few decades. Lymphadenopathy and lymphocytosis occasionally develop with phenytoin administration, but these are benign [3]. This pseudolymphoma abates when treatment is stopped. Much more difficult to reverse and manage are severe immunologic problems, such as Stevens-Johnson syndrome and exfoliative dermatitis [8].

Psychiatric problems are less likely to occur with phenytoin use than are neurologic reactions, but the range of psychiatric problems that occur is broad [7, 9, 10]. Many patients complain of intellectual slowing and impaired concentration, at least when they first start taking the medication. Rarely, patients have tactile or visual hallucinations [11]. If the individual has minor problems with intellectual function before phenytoin is introduced, confusion and disorientation may be prominent when the patient is taking therapeutic doses of the antiepileptic [10]. Some patients have problems with their memory or their ability to calculate; families and friends often notice that the patient is more irascibile on the drug than off [7]. In many cases in which psychological disturbances are prominent, the problem is toxic interactions with other drugs taken in conjunction with the phenytoin. With any change in intellectual function or affect, the serum phenytoin level should be checked. Excessively high serum phenytoin levels may increase seizure frequency [12].

Hyperglycemia occasionally develops with phenytoin use [5]. This is apparently caused by the ability of this drug to inhibit insulin release from the pancreas [5]. Although the effect usually is fairly subtle, patients who are borderline diabetics may become symptomatic for diabetes mellitus after they take phenytoin [5]. An additional endocrinologic effect of this drug is to increase the catabolism of thyroid hormones [13]. The patient with normal thyroid function will compensate automatically. The patient on thyroid supplements because of hypothyroidism will require an increase in the thyroid hormone dose to avoid worsening hypothyroidism.

Complications of Long-term Use

With long-term phenytoin use (oral use for more than a decade), the patient may develop minor peripheral nerve damage that causes an annoying, but not particularly disabling, peripheral neuropathy. On examination, the patient may have little more than absent reflexes, but the neuropathy may be more obviously manifested as paresthesias. A relative folate deficiency, induced in some people by chronic phenytoin use, may play a role in the development of this peripheral neuropathy, but there is no evidence that folate supplements prevent this neuropathy. No treatment is known.

Another problem that develops after years of antiepileptic use and that is probably related to phenytoin is cerebellar damage. This causes truncal ataxia and may be related to a drug-induced folate deficiency [14]. Cerebellar damage is seen most often in patients taking very high doses of several antiepileptic drugs for many years and is associated with fairly high serum levels of phenobarbital [14]. Whether the damage is caused by phenytoin, phenobarbital, or combinations of antiepileptics working together is unresolved.

Drug Interactions

Several drugs affect the rate at which phenytoin is metabolized and the percent of the drug that is bound to serum proteins. A variety of widely used psychoactive drugs interfere with the metabolism of phenytoin, including diazepam (Valium), chlorpromazine (Thorazine), prochlorperazine (Compazine), methylphenidate hydrochloride (Ritalin), and chlordiazepoxide hydrochloride (Librium) [14]. Some drugs increase the effective serum level of phenytoin if the patient takes the drugs chronically [15]. These include cimetidine, isoniazid, disulfiram, chloramphenicol, sulfamethizole, phenylbutazone, warfarin, ethosuximide, and estrogens.

Phenytoin lowers serum folate levels and interferes with the metabolism of vitamins K and D. This interference may be substantial enough to pose problems for women on phenytoin during childbirth, but the incidence of bleeding during pregnancy in women on any type of antiepileptic is the same as that for women not on antiepileptic drugs [8, 16]. As noted in Chapter 8, pregnant women who do take phenytoin should be given supplementary vitamin K for several months before delivery, and their newborns should receive vitamin K at birth [8].

Fetal Hydantoin Syndrome

Children born to women on phenytoin often exhibit lower birth weights, smaller head circumferences, and slower growth and development. As discussed in Chapter 8, some of the offspring of women who take antiepileptic drugs during their pregnancies have birth defects, which include abnormal facial features, cardiac defects, and nail and digital hypoplasia. Some children have mental retardation as well as poor physical development. These problems were initially recognized as a syndrome in the offspring of women taking phenytoin and were consequently called the *fetal hydantoin syndrome,* because phenytoin (diphenylhydantoin) belongs to the hydantoin family of drugs [17].

The assumption has been that the phenytoin has deleterious effects on the fetus that may produce developmental defects or delays. More experience with women on other antiepileptics and with women not on antiepileptics suggests that the specificity of phenytoin in producing this syndrome may have been overstated [18]. Women on anticonvulsants other than phenytoin have offspring with the same skeletal and developmental problems as those found in the fetal hydantoin syndrome, and the children most often exhibiting the abnormalities are those exposed to multiple antiepileptic drugs during gestation (see Chapter 8).

PHENOBARBITAL

Phenobarbital is one of the oldest anticonvulsants in use, but it is not routinely preferred to treat any adult seizure disorder other than status epilepticus (Fig. 14–3). It is the drug of choice for complex febrile seizures and neonatal seizures, but even in these situations, it should be replaced by another antiepileptic as the child matures if the seizures persist and assume a more specific pattern [3]. It is used in children because it is easily absorbed and well tolerated, but it is also widely used in adults because it is familiar to most physicians. Generalized tonic-clonic, simple partial, and complex partial seizure usually respond to phenobarbital, but sedation and behavioral disturbances induced by the drug have increasingly limited its use as less toxic drugs have been developed [3, 8].

Phenobarbital can be given orally as a tablet or syrup or by injection intravenously or intramuscularly. An intrarectal solution also is well absorbed and sometimes helpful with infants who have upper gastrointestinal problems, such as vomiting. The peak serum level is not reached until 12 to 18 hours after an oral dose, even when absorption by that route is excellent [4]. When it is used at high doses by any route, breathing must be monitored.

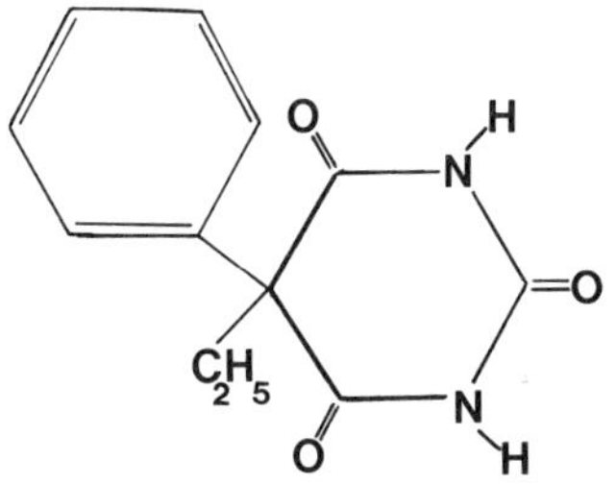

Figure 14–3.
Chemical structure of phenobarbital.

Most adults achieve a therapeutic drug level of 15 to 35 µg/ml on a regular oral dose of 100 to 200 mg daily [3]. Children reach therapeutic levels with 3 to 5 mg/kg/day. Infants may require more. As with phenytoin, serum levels must be monitored closely in neonates and very young infants, because metabolism of the phenobarbital is unpredictable in these very small children.

Phenobarbital has many adverse effects, but most are dose-related. It may make generalized absence seizures more frequent in children given this drug inappropriately [8]. Some children become hyperactive, aggressive, and tearful [11]. Such hyperactive children have reduced attention spans and are easily distracted and very destructive.

Most adults have no adverse reactions to phenobarbital except for mild sedation until toxic levels are reached. With toxicity, the adult exhibits a staggering gait, slurred speech, and nystagmus [11]. Patients with serum phenobarbital levels of more than 60 µg/ml usually become disoriented and confused, but this is so much in excess of the therapeutic range that the patient usually is ataxic or heavily sedated first [4, 11].

The catabolism of phenobarbital is different at different ages. Estimates of drug half-lives for this and other antiepileptics must be considered reliable only for the average healthy young adult, unless otherwise indicated (Table 14–2). Because the elderly adult metabolizes phenobarbital more slowly or because his nervous system is less resilient than that of the young adult, he is more vulnerable to the side effects of phenobarbital than is the young adult. This increased sensitivity usually is manifested as restlessness, confusion, and severe depression at fairly low serum levels of the antiepileptic.

Abrupt phenobarbital withdrawal causes seizures even in patients not previously known to have seizures. An additional disadvantage of phenobarbital is that it is used as a recreational drug by some individuals. Alternatively, some patients may take a large number of pills in a suicide attempt. The number of pills that must be taken to suppress breathing varies from patient to patient, but a successful suicide is very possible with phenobarbital. With unsuccessful suicide attempts, toxic effects of the phenobarbital may abate

Table 14–2.
Characteristics of Common Antiepileptic Drugs

Drug	Serum Half-life (hours)		Protein Binding (%)
	Child	Adult	
Phenytoin	3–11	22–40	88–92
Carbamazepine	6–16	8–19	67–81
Valproic acid	4–14	7–17	90–95
Ethosuximide	24–30	50–60	—
Primidone	6–8	8–16	0–20
Phenobarbital	30–50	50–96	50
Clonazepam	16–60	16–60	—

only after several weeks [9, 11]. The number and magnitude of adverse reactions associated with this drug also lead to a high level of noncompliance. Approximately 20 percent of the patients advised to take phenobarbital either do not take it at all or do not take it as recommended [9].

PRIMIDONE

Primidone (Mysoline) is closely related to phenobarbital structurally, and it is partly metabolized to phenobarbital after absorption (Fig. 14–4). Primidone and its metabolic products, phenobarbital and phenylethylmalonamide, are all effective antiepileptics [8]. Many physicians consider primidone the drug of choice for the management of complex partial seizures, and even those who prefer carbamazepine recognize it as a valuable alternative drug for the treatment of this type of epilepsy [4]. Generalized tonic-clonic seizures and complex febrile convulsions are also sensitive to primidone [4, 19].

Primidone is widely available as a tablet or syrup and can be used by both children and adults. It can be taken orally, intramuscularly, or intravenously. A therapeutic level of 6 to 12 µg/ml can usually be reached with an oral dose of 750 to 1,500 mg daily for an adult or 10 to 25 mg/kg/day for a child [3, 11]. Because it is metabolized in part to phenobarbital, any routine check of the serum drug level should include a measurement of the serum phenobarbital level. A patient who appears toxic with a low serum primidone level may have a toxic phenobarbital level, which will account for the symptoms.

Toxic effects include sedation, nausea, and gait ataxia [3]. More idiosyncratic reactions to this drug include acute confusional states, loss of libido, impotence, impaired concentration, and persecutory delusions [8, 9, 11]. It is contraindicated in some patients with porphyria [8].

One advantage of primidone is that the peak serum level is reached within only 3 hours of an oral dose, but this also means that toxic manifestations of a primidone dose appear much sooner than with phenobarbital [4]. Many of the toxic effects of primidone, especially the sedation, can be minimized by starting the patient on a low dose, such as 125 mg three times daily, and increasing it over the course of 2 to 3 weeks.

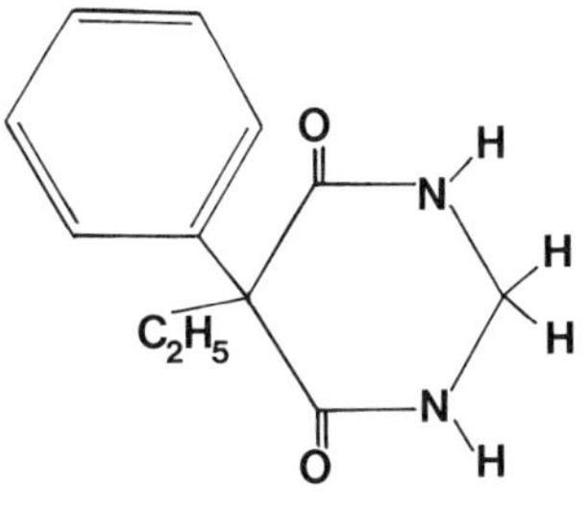

Figure 14–4.
Chemical structure of primidone.

CARBAMAZEPINE

Carbamazepine (Tegretol) is believed by many physicians to be the drug of choice for complex partial seizures, and it is a useful alternative drug for the management of simple partial and generalized tonic-clonic seizures [4, 9, 12]. That it has substantial advantages in complex partial epilepsy over alternative medication, such as primidone, is not well established, but it is at least as good as any other drug currently available for the treatment of this type of epilepsy.

Carbamazepine can be given to children or adults. It usually is taken orally as a 200 mg tablet. Because of gastrointestinal irritation associated with the drug, most patients must start with only half a tablet (100 mg) two or three times daily and increase the dosage to a therapeutic level over the course of 2 to 4 weeks. In most adults, 600 to 1,200 mg daily will produce a therapeutic serum level of 6 to 10 μg/ml (see Table 12-3) [3]. Children may require 20 to 30 mg/kg/day to maintain the same therapeutic level [3].

When carbamazepine was first introduced, several reports indicated that thrombocytopenia was a fairly common side effect. Its incidence subsequently proved to be greatly exaggerated, but some individuals do develop thrombocytopenia and others develop a reversible leukopenia as an idiosyncratic reaction to the drug [8]. The most frequently observed toxic reactions are neurologic and gastrointestinal [12]. Patients often develop heartburn or indigestion when they first start on the drug, but this passes within days or weeks even if the patient's dose is increased. Vertigo, dizziness, and diplopia develop in many patients with excessively high serum levels of carbamazepine [4, 11]. Paresthesias and fatigue that persist for days after the drug is stopped may develop in some patients.

Although carbamazepine does not, as a rule, exacerbate seizure activity, rare patients have idiosyncratic reactions that include an acute increase in seizure frequency [12]. This acute aberrant reaction is especially likely in children with minor motor seizures [12]. If such a reaction occurs, it will end when use of the drug is stopped. Drug interactions usually are more important in the exacerbation of seizures than is any aberrant reaction to carbamazepine. Even if the additional drug is itself an antiepileptic, it may decrease the serum level or effectiveness of carbamazepine. Phenytoin and valproic acid in particular routinely depress the serum level of carbamazepine if they are given concurrently (see Table 12–4). Any patient taking a combination of antiepileptic drugs should have the levels of all drugs checked regularly, which may range from every 6 months for the totally asymptomatic individual to every week for the toxic or poorly controlled patient.

ETHOSUXIMIDE

Ethosuximide (Zarontin) is the drug of choice in generalized absence (petit mal) epilepsy, especially when the patient has classic 3-Hz spike-and-wave

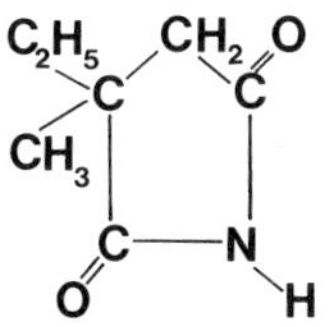

Figure 14–5.
Chemical structure of ethosuximide.

absence attacks unassociated with generalized tonic-clonic seizures (Fig. 14–5) [8, 9]. Methsuximide (Celontin) is a closely related drug that is the first-choice alternative for individuals who cannot tolerate ethosuximide. Unfortunately, a child allergic to ethosuximide will usually be allergic to methsuximide as well. Both of these drugs are used almost exclusively in children, because the types of epilepsy in which they are most effective are seen most often in children. Of course, they can be used for adults with seizure combinations that are poorly responsive to other antiepileptic drugs.

Ethosuximide usually is given orally as a tablet or syrup, but preparations for rectal administration are available. The drug is quickly absorbed, within 2 to 4 hours after an oral dose, and the serum level usually stabilizes within a week of initiating treatment with a maintenance dose [8]. Therapeutic serum levels of 50 to 100 μg/ml usually are maintained with oral doses of 20 to 40 mg/kg/day in children [3, 11] (see Table 12–3). Adults generally require 750 to 2,000 mg daily to achieve therapeutic serum levels [3].

Adverse reactions include gastrointestinal upset, night terrors, agitation, and paranoid delusions [8, 11]. All of these are idiosyncratic and unrelated to the dose taken [8]. Rashes and thrombocytopenia occur in some individuals. Mood disturbances occasionally develop and range from extreme apathy and lack of initiative to unfounded euphoria [11]. The patients most at risk for developing paranoia or destructive behavior as an adverse reaction to the drug are those with long-standing intellectual impairment [11].

VALPROIC ACID

Valproic (dipropylacetic) acid (Depakene, Epilim) has a structure different from all other antiepileptics (Fig. 14–6). It is a branched-chain, eight-carbon fatty acid, of which the sodium salt, valproate sodium, is marketed as a liquid for patients who cannot take tablets of valproic acid [20]. Many physicians recommend this as the drug of choice for benign juvenile myoclonic epilepsy, and it is a first-line alternative for several other types of epilepsy (see Table 12–2) [8, 21].

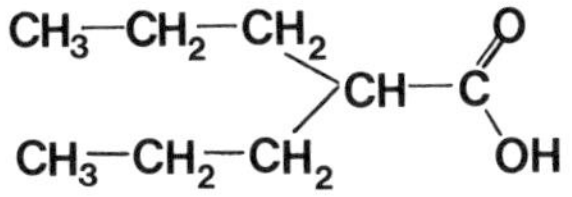

Figure 14–6.
Chemical structure of valproic acid.

It is very effective against generalized tonic-clonic and absence seizures and is useful in the management of myoclonic photosensitive epilepsy, complex febrile convulsions, and absence seizures associated with generalized tonic-clonic seizures [3, 5, 8, 19]. Although ethosuximide causes less gastrointestinal distress than valproic acid and is at least as effective against absence seizures, valproic acid may be a better drug for those patients with both generalized absence and tonic-clonic seizures because it is highly effective against both, whereas ethosuximide is not very useful in managing tonic-clonic seizures [20].

Valproic acid is available as either a tablet or a syrup and has recently been released as a slow-release preparation (Depakote) that requires fewer daily doses to maintain a therapeutic serum level. Given alone, a dose of 15 to 18 mg/kg/day usually is enough to produce a therapeutic serum level in a child, but when valproic acid is given with other anticonvulsants, its protein binding and rate of metabolism often are affected, and doses of 18 to 25 mg/kg/day may be needed [5, 8].

Phenytoin, phenobarbital, and carbamazepine all lower the serum level of valproic acid by inducing liver enzymes that speed up the catabolism of valproic acid (see Table 12–4) [5]. Oral dosages of 1 to 3 g (four to twelve tablets) per day usually will produce a therapeutic serum level of 50 to 100 µg/ml in an adult [3]. Three to four doses of medication usually provide an adequately stable serum level to ensure good seizure control. One or two doses of the slow-release preparation are equally effective. The dosage required in children is much more variable, and serum levels of the drug should dictate the dose given [3].

The commonest adverse reactions to valproic acid are gastrointestinal disturbances. Up to 50 percent of the patients who take this drug complain of anorexia, nausea, vomiting, or disturbing changes in bowel patterns [20]. These are usually transient and can often be minimized by giving the drug along with meals. Children are more likely than adults to have gastrointestinal complaints.

Most adults will first develop signs of toxicity at total daily dosages greater than 2.5 g [8]. This will often be limited to sedation, but some will develop thrombocytopenia, increased platelet aggregation, hypofibrinogenemia, or elevated hepatic enzyme levels [8, 22]. Hair loss occurs in up to 4 percent of patients using valproic acid, but this distressing problem generally is transient, even though it may not appear until the patient has been on the drug for 3 or 4 months [20]. Despite the gastrointestinal disturbances associated with valproic acid, some patients complain of weight gain after they have taken the drug for several months.

Neurologic reactions include tremors, headache, bed-wetting, insomnia, and anorexia. Most of these adverse reactions clear within hours or days when drug use is stopped. Some patients given valproic acid and clonazepam together have developed absence status epilepticus, but it has not been established whether this was necessarily a result of the drugs' interaction [20]. Obviously, physicians would be wise to avoid this drug combination.

Lethal hepatic dysfunctions have occurred in rare patients taking valproic acid for 3 days to 6 months, and the basis for this adverse reaction is still unknown [3, 8]. Apparently, it is not dose-related and usually occurs in association with congenital malformations, mental retardation, or other types of organic brain disease [8]. Minor disturbances of hepatic enzymes are as common with phenytoin as they are with valproic acid, and so these may not be helpful markers of the patient's susceptibility to serious liver damage with use of this medication [5]. Because valproic acid is remarkably effective against several different types of generalized and partial seizures, it will probably see much wider use if the basis for its more dangerous side effects can be determined.

BENZODIAZEPINES

Benzodiazepines have limited usefulness as anticonvulsants, but there are some notable exceptions. Diazepam is extremely effective for short periods when administered intravenously to treat status epilepticus (see Chapter 13). Lorazepam has occasionally been useful in managing patients with tonic-clonic or absence status epilepticus. Chlordiazepoxide and oxazepam are not used as antiepileptics.

Paradoxical effects are occasionally seen with these drugs. For instance, benzodiazepines given intravenously to children with Lennox-Gastaut syndrome may precipitate tonic status epilepticus [12]. Whenever benzodiazepines are given to a patient with epilepsy, it is important to remember that the catabolism of the drugs will be affected by old age, hepatic disease, and interactions with other drugs such as estrogens, cimetidine, disulfiram, and isoniazid [23].

Diazepam

Diazepam (Valium) is not effective orally as an antiepileptic drug, but it is very effective when given intramuscularly or intravenously. It is most often used to manage status epilepticus, in which case it is given intravenously in 10 mg doses. The dose usually is repeated every 10 to 15 minutes until the seizure activity stops, up to a maximum dose of 50 mg in the adult. The main disadvantage of the drug is that antiepileptic levels are not sustained in the blood and so another anticonvulsant must be given along with the diazepam to keep the status epilepticus from recurring.

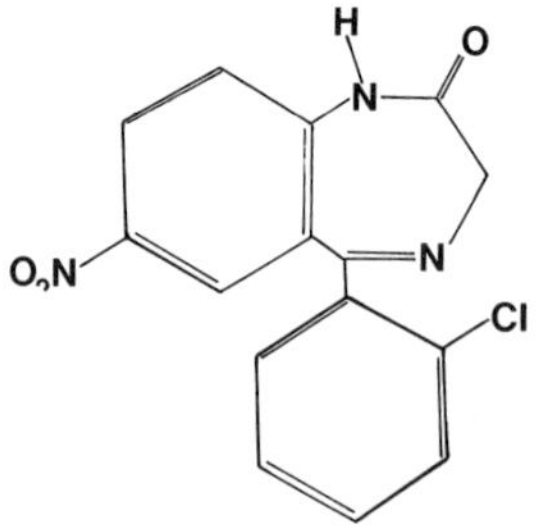

Figure 14–7.
Chemical structure of clonazepam.

Clonazepam

Clonazepam (Clonopin) is an effective oral antiepileptic drug for several types of seizure disorders, but it is used primarily for the management of myoclonic and akinetic seizures (Fig. 14–7) [3, 15]. Some physicians use it intermittently to manage simple febrile seizures, but there is controversy regarding whether these should be treated at all [19].

Clonazepam is used as an alternative drug for absence seizures when other medications have failed, but it is associated with many behavioral side effects in children [24]. These include irritability, aggressiveness, emotional instability, and hyperactivity [25]. Drowsiness and ataxia are more common adverse effects [3, 24]. These are apparently dose-related and may disappear with fairly small adjustments in the dosage. More idiosyncratic reactions include excessive salivation and bronchial secretion, problems that occasionally interfere with use of the drug in children [24].

A therapeutic serum level of 13 to 72 ng/ml can usually be reached with an oral dosage of 1.5 to 2.0 mg daily in an adult [3]. Clonazepam is widely available as 0.5-, 1-, or 2-mg tablets. Side effects usually are obvious at a serum level greater than 72 ng/ml, and so the range between therapeutic and toxic levels is very narrow [25]. Children can usually tolerate 0.01 to 0.02 mg/kg/day orally [3].

Drug interactions must be watched for carefully with this drug. Using it in combination with valproic acid increases the risk of generalized seizures [3]. Patients on high doses of clonazepam for several weeks should be tapered off the drug to avoid withdrawal seizures.

Lorazepam

Lorazepam (Ativan) has been used in some patients to manage tonic-clonic status epilepticus, but it is not widely accepted as an anticonvulsant on a daily basis. A single intravenous dose of lorazepam, 0.1 mg/kg may suffice to stop the seizure activity in the patient with status epilepticus, but another antiepileptic with a longer serum half-life, such as phenytoin, should also be given to prevent the recurrence of seizures during the subsequent few hours.

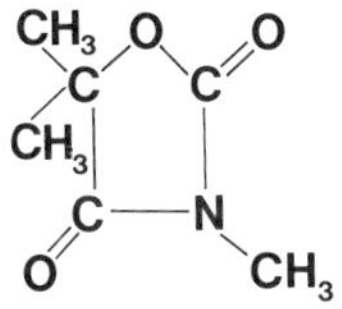

Figure 14–8.
Chemical structure of trimethadione.

Lorazepam is available in 1-mg tablets that are widely prescribed to relieve anxiety and insomnia. At an oral dose of 1 mg twice daily, it is an alternative to other antiepileptics for patients with complex partial epilepsy. The main disadvantage of the drug is the high incidence of drowsiness associated with a therapeutic dose.

TRIMETHADIONE

In the past, trimethadione was popular as an alternative medication for the control of generalized absence seizures, but the development of safer drugs has reduced its use considerably (Fig. 14–8). Adults usually tolerate 900 to 2,100 mg of drug daily; children require 10 to 25 mg/kg/day [15]. The therapeutic level ranges from 6 to 41 μg/ml, and the plasma half-life of the drug is 12 to 24 hours [15].

Adverse reactions include headache, photophobia, irritability, and rashes. Some idiosyncratic hematologic reactions occur with this drug, and some patients have a lupus-like reaction. Women of childbearing age should not be exposed to the drug, because there is a very high incidence of birth defects associated with its use.

ADRENOCORTICOTROPIC HORMONE

Adrenocorticotropic hormone is useful as an antiepileptic agent in the management of infantile spasms (see Chapter 13). It has no application with any other type of epilepsy. Although the adverse effects associated with this agent are substantial, there is no equally effective alternative for infantile spasms. Adverse effects include an increased susceptibility to infections, sleep disturbances, hypertension, moon facies, and hyperglycemia. This hormone is never used for more than a few months in these infants. Its long-term effects have not been determined.

OTHER DRUGS USED FOR SEIZURE CONTROL

Several other drugs have been used to control seizures in various settings, but most have no current applications. Acetazolamide (Diamox) was long considered a valuable adjunct in the treatment of generalized absence seizures, but much more clearly effective drugs have replaced it [26]. Triple bromide salts are still used occasionally for children who fail to respond to other antiepileptic drugs, but the sedation and acne caused by these bromides make them a last-choice alternative. Acetylureas such as pheneturide and phenacemide are effective against some types of complex partial seizures, but they are not as well tolerated as carbamazepine or primidone. Life-threatening reactions in some patients have made them unpopular for routine use. Some obstetricians have favored various magnesium sulfate preparations for treating seizures in eclampsia, but more conventional antiepileptics, such as phenytoin or phenobarbital, are more effective and less likely to cause electrolyte problems.

With intractable seizures, a variety of intravenous regimens have been devised that may suppress the seizure activity but probably simply anesthetize the patient in most cases. The most clearly antiepileptic preparation is a 2% paraldehyde solution. This is used primarily for tonic-clonic status epilepticus that has failed to respond to other medications. The solution is infused at a rate adequate to suppress all clinical signs of seizure activity without producing a fluid overload (see Chapter 13). The solution must be shielded from light because it is very unstable, and many of the plastic intravenous tubes used to deliver fluids will dissolve with protracted exposure to paraldehyde.

A lidocaine hydrochloride infusion is simpler to use than a paraldehyde drip, but lidocaine is less clearly an antiepileptic than an anesthetic agent. Cardiovascular monitoring of any patient given intravenous lidocaine is appropriate, but most patients can tolerate up to 200 mg of the drug over the course of 2 hours. This may not be an adequate dose to suppress the clinical seizure activity, but higher doses are only appropriate when the patient's condition is life-threatening.

General anesthetics, such as halothane, may be appropriate when the patient has profound tonic-clonic activity leading to substantial muscle destruction and hyperthermia. The anesthetic will not stop the seizure activity, but it may reduce the risk of physiologic problems, such as renal failure, that often are lethal in the rare cases of status epilepticus that cannot be managed with other drugs.

REFERENCES

1. Rodin, E.A. *The Prognosis of Patients with Epilepsy.* Springfield, Ill.: Charles C Thomas, 1968.
2. Merritt, H.H., Putnam T.J. Sodium diphenyl hydantoinate in treatment of convulsive disorders. *J.A.M.A.* 111:1068–1073, 1938.
3. Drugs for epilepsy, *Med. Lett. Drugs Ther.* 25(643):81–84, 1983.
4. Penry, J.K., Newmark, M.E. The use of antiepileptic drugs. *Ann. Intern. Med.* 90:207, 1979.

5. Wilder, B.J., Ramsay, R.E., Murphy, J.V., et al. Comparison of valproic acid and phenytoin in newly diagnosed tonic-clonic seizures. *Neurology* (N.Y.) 33(11):1474–1476, 1983.

6. Kang, H., Leppik, I.E. Phenytoin binding and renal transplantation. *Neurology* (N.Y.) 34(11):83–85, 1984.

7. McLain, L.W., Martin, J.T., Allen, J.H. Cerebellar degeneration due to chronic phenytoin therapy. *Ann. Neurol.* 7:18, 1980.

8. Delgado-Escueta, A.V., Treiman, D.M., Walsh, G.O. The treatable epilepsies (part 2). *N. Engl. J. Med.* 308(26):1576–1584, 1983.

9. Booker, H.E. Management of the difficult patient with complex partial seizures. *Adv. Neurol.* 11:369, 1975.

10. Franks, R.E., Richter, A.J. Schizophrenia-like psychosis associated with anticonvulsant toxicity. *Am. J. Psychiatry* 136:973, 1979.

11. Tollefson, G. Psychiatric implications of anticonvulsant drugs. *J. Clin. Psychiatry* 41:295, 1980.

12. Shields, W.D., Saslow, E. Myoclonic, atonic, and absence seizures following institution of carbamazepine in children. *Neurology* (N.Y.) 33(11):1487–1489, 1983.

13. Drug interactions update. *Med. Lett. Drugs Ther.* 26(654):11–14, 1984.

14. Muñoz-Garcia, D., Del Ser, T., Bermejo, F., Portera, A. Truncal ataxia in chronic anticonvulsant treatment: association with drug-induced folate deficiency. *J. Neurol. Sci.* 55(3):305–311, 1982.

15. *Drugs of Choice.* New Rochelle, N.Y.: The Medical Letter. 1977, pp. 45–63.

16. Nelson, K.B., Ellenberg, J.H. Maternal seizure disorder, outcome of pregnancy, and neurologic abnormalities in the children. *Neurology* (N.Y.) 32(11):1247–1254, 1982.

17. Hanson, J.W., Smith, D.W. The fetal hydantoin syndrome. *J. Pediatr.* 87:285–290, 1975.

18. Granstrom, M.L., Hiilesmaa, V.K. Malformations and minor anomalies in the children of epileptic mothers: preliminary results of the prospective Helsinki study. In Jans, D., Dam, M., Richens, A., et al. (eds.), *Epilepsy, Pregnancy, and the Child.* New York: Raven Press, 1982, pp. 303–307.

19. Herranz, J.L., Armijo, J.A., Arteaga, R. Effectiveness and toxicity of phenobarbital, primidone, and sodium valproate in the prevention of febrile convulsions, controlled by plasma levels. *Epilepsia* 25(1):89–95, 1984.

20. Browne, T.R. Valproic acid. *N. Engl. J. Med.* 302(12):661–665, 1980.

21. Asconape, J., Penry, J.K. Some clinical and EEG aspects of benign juvenile myoclonic epilepsy. *Epilepsia* 25(1):108–114, 1984.

22. Bruni, J., Wilder, B.J. Valproic acid. *Arch. Neurol.* 36:393, 1979.

23. Greenblatt, D.J., Shader, R.I., Abernathy, D.R. Current status of benzodiazepines (part 1). *N. Engl. J. Med.* 309(6):354–358, 1983.

24. Browne, T.R. Clonazepam. *N. Engl. J. Med.* 299:812, 1978.

25. Stahl, Y., Persson, A., Petters, I., et al. Kinetics of clonazepam in relation to electroencephalographic and clinical effects. *Epilepsia* 24(2):225–231, 1983.

26. Millichap, J.G. Drug treatment of convulsive disorders. *N. Engl. J. Med.* 286(9):464–469, 1972.

15. Nonpharmaceutical Approaches to Treatment

Antiepileptic drugs are the best treatment currently available for epilepsy. As with any therapeutic regimen, there will be patients who do not respond or who are dissatisfied with the demands of the treatment itself. With epilepsy, the proportion of patients who are unhappy with the results or demands of the drugs used is substantial. Reassuring the patients that new drugs are being tested and introduced every year may do little to allay their frustration and pessimism. Even the medications that are available are far from ideal, that ideal being a medication that can be taken infrequently and still suppress the seizures while causing no adverse reactions. All of these considerations prompt patients to seek nonpharmaceutical treatment measures.

Patients whose seizures are well controlled often look for simpler therapies, and simpler often means unorthodox. This willingness to try unscientific treatment modalities is encouraged by fragmented reports of miraculous recoveries. Folk remedies, such as vitamin regimens, spinal manipulation, faith healing, holy water, and special diets, have irrepressible popularity, even though their effectiveness generally is negligible, whereas the harm done to patients who place confidence in these remedies may be appreciable.

Of course, there are nonpharmaceutical adjuncts to treatment that do help some individuals. Brain surgery clearly improves the outlook for some individuals, but it is a drastic step that yields its best results with a highly motivated patient [1]. Less drastic measures, such as electrical stimulation of the brain and dietary management of seizures, have been experimented with for many years with little success.

Group therapy and rehabilitation are valuable adjuncts to any type of epilepsy treatment when seizure control is poor. Group therapy involving the families of epileptic individuals is especially likely to minimize the stress faced by the individual with poorly controlled seizures [2]. Rehabilitation helps get the patient back to work and more involved with those around him. Encouragement and assistance that aid patients in resuming a more normal life have antiepileptic effects of their own.

SURGERY

Surgical removal of a focus of abnormal electrical activity in the brain is occasionally effective in controlling epilepsy that could not be controlled with medication [3, 4]. Since any operation on the brain may produce a new seizure focus, removal of brain tissue to control seizure activity is performed only as a last resort. An alternative to removing the irritable brain tissue is isolating it from much of the cortex. Both of these approaches are currently used in the surgical management of intractable epilepsy.

Patients who are appropriately considered candidates for this type of intervention must have been tried on optional antiepileptic medication [5]. Surgery is neither simpler nor safer than medication, and so it should not be considered an alternative to medical treatment. If the patient has had adequate trials with appropriate medications alone and in combination over the course of several years and has had little or no relief from seizures, then an operation should be considered [5].

Good surgical candidates exhibit the following characteristics:

Normal intelligence quotient
High level of motivation
No diffuse brain damage
No generalized seizures
Clearly defined seizure focus
Seizures that were uncontrolled by medication for more than 4 years
Seizure focus that is resectable without causing major neurologic deficits
Complex partial seizures starting with motionless staring

Many patients chosen for surgical treatment have taken antiepileptic drugs with no success for more than a decade; attempts at controlling seizures with medication alone should be abandoned only after a minimum of 3 to 4 years of drug trials [1].

It is also important that the seizures be of such frequency and severity that they substantially interfere with the patient's life [5]. If a fairly mild seizure occurs a few times per month, the patient may be annoyed and frustrated enough to consider seizure surgery, but he should not be considered an appropriate candidate. Most patients with diffuse brain damage or a long-standing psychosis do not profit from the surgery, and so they, too, should not be considered surgical candidates. A notable exception is the patient with a structural lesion in the temporal lobe that is believed to be contributing to the psychosis as well as to the seizure disorder [6].

Surgical resection of a seizure focus is only feasible when a distinct region of abnormal activity can be localized in the brain either by electroencephalography or direct recording of electrical activity at the surface of the brain [3, 7]. In addition, removal of the brain tissue wherein lies the abnormal activity must not cause an unacceptable neurologic deficit [5]. Care must be taken to exclude patients who will have impaired memory if a temporal lobe focus is resected or impaired speech if a frontal lobe focus is removed.

Those least likely to benefit from surgical intervention include individuals with intelligence quotient scores lower than 75 or bilateral neurologic deficits [1]. Highly motivated patients do better than ambivalent ones, and chances for a good result are best if the individual has a highly circumscribed anterior temporal lobe lesion [8]. Patients with bilateral electroencephalographic abnormalities on routine recordings or clinical evidence of generalized seizures do much more poorly after surgery than patients with unilateral foci associated with complex partial seizures [5].

Preoperative Studies

Highly invasive electroencephalographic studies are appropriate in preparation for seizure surgery. That a focus exists and the precise location of that focus must be determined with a probable error limited to less than 1 or 2 cm. In many cases, this requires studies involving nasopharyngeal and sphenoidal leads. In most centers where this kind of operation is performed, preliminary recordings from the surface and deep in the brain are used to better define the seizure focus. Electrodes are placed in the brain only for a preoperative study: It is assumed that the cortex damaged by the electrodes will be largely removed during the resection if surgical intervention appears to be advisable [7].

Extensive neuropsychological studies are done routinely before and after the operation to determine which intellectual functions, if any, are impaired or improved by the operation. These types of studies provide objective indicators of the patient's progress after the operation, and they provide insight into what the patient's abilities and disabilities will be [9].

Internal carotid infusion of amobarbital sodium (Wada Test) will help determine whether memory will be impaired after resection of one temporal lobe. This fast-acting barbiturate transiently interferes with function in the infused temporal lobe and thereby unmasks deficits, especially in memory, likely to develop with resection of the impaired lobe [1]. The amobarbital infusion also will reveal whether the nondominant hemisphere is truly nondominant for speech. If the seizure focus appears to be in the right frontal lobe near the region homologous to Broca's speech area, the barbiturate infusion will establish that removal of the cortex near the seizure focus will not produce an expressive aphasia [10]. Any resection performed on the speech-dominant temporal lobe is routinely limited to the anterior portion of that lobe as part of a concerted effort to avoid injury to the posterior third of the superior temporal gyrus, an injury that could produce a receptive aphasia [11].

Temporal Lobe Surgery

Temporal lobe surgery for seizure control has most often been employed in cases of complex partial seizures originating in the temporal lobe. The seizures in approximately 60 percent of patients with complex partial epilepsy are inadequately controlled with medication [12]. Surgery is an attractive option for the individual whose seizure focus is in the temporal lobe, because the anterior part of the temporal lobe usually can be resected with little apparent neurologic deficit [3, 4]. The proportion of patients having complex partial seizures with temporal lobe foci who have failed to improve on medication and who would probably improve with an operation is controversial, but the estimates run as high as 1 of every 3 such patients [12].

The procedure routinely involves resection of the anterior 5 to 6 cm of the abnormal temporal lobe. The uncus, hippocampus, and amygdala are resected along with other temporal lobe structures [1]. These structures are situated deep inside and along the mesial aspect of the temporal lobe. The area involved is free of motor pathways, but a visual field cut may remain as a permanent consequence of the surgery, because part of the optic radiation from the lateral geniculate travels anteriorly in the temporal lobe before turning laterally and posteriorly to reach the occipital lobe.

Gyrectomy

Well-defined seizure foci do occur outside the temporal lobe, and many occur in relatively "silent" areas of the cerebral cortex. Once the lesion has been delineated with electrical recordings from the surface of the cortex, the abnormal gyrus or gyri can be resected (see Fig. 2–5). The better the preoperative resolution of the seizure focus, the better will be the results of such a gyrectomy. Highly specialized techniques, such as positron emission tomography, may help to define the seizure focus, but in all patients, the clinical signs, electroencephalographic records, and computed tomographic evidence of focal pathology should be considered before any surgery is performed.

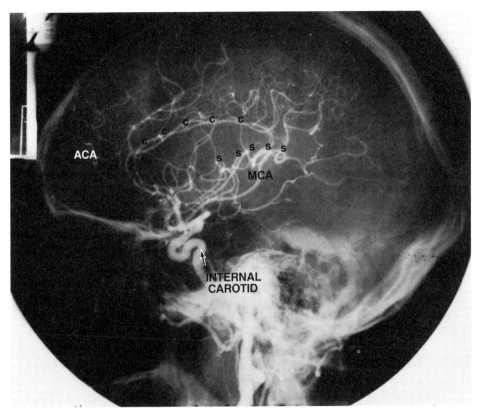

Figure 15–1.
The pericallosal branches (c) of the anterior cerebral artery outline the anterior corpus callosum above which they lie. The middle cerebral artery (MCA) similarly defines the sylvian fissure by looping over the temporal lobe with its sylvian branches (s).

Corpus Callosum Section

Severing the corpus callosum, the principal white matter connection between the cerebral hemispheres, is performed much less frequently than temporal lobe resection or selective removal of part of a cerebral gyrus, but occasionally it is useful [13]. It is assumed that cutting the corpus callosum isolates seizure activity to one hemisphere and thereby limits its spread (Fig. 15–1). Supporting this assumption is the observed decrease in seizure frequency and severity in individuals who undergo the procedure. The type of epilepsy exhibited by the patient does not change after the surgery, but seizures that previously generalized will be much less likely to spread. The entire corpus callosum need not be cut to obtain the maximum benefit from this procedure. Most surgeons limit the incision to the anterior two-thirds of the callosum and spare the splenium corporis callosi.

Results

The results with any of these surgical procedures are greatly influenced by the types of patients selected for operation. Defining *morbidity* after the operation is difficult, because the nature of the procedure guarantees that there will be something different about the patient after he is surgically treated. With corpus callosum section, the patient exhibits peculiar psychological features attributed to a split-brain injury [14]. With a selective gyrus resection, gaze disturbances, constructional problems, mild apraxias, or other nondisabling neurologic deficits may appear postoperatively.

What can be defined most confidently after surgery are the mortality and rate of seizure remission. Mortality for anterior temporal lobectomy is negligible in competent hands, and morbidity runs at approximately 2 percent [1]. Morbidity is lowest for individuals undergoing right (nondominant) temporal lobe resection.

Complex partial seizures stop after anterior temporal lobectomy in 60 to 80 percent of the patients subjected to surgery, but antiepileptic drugs still may be needed to fully suppress seizure activity postoperatively. Probably because not all complex partial seizures originate in the anterior temporal lobe, there are some patients who do not respond to this procedure [5]. Of some predictive value is the character of the clinical seizure before any invasive techniques are used. Patients with complex partial seizures that begin with motionless staring, sterotyped automatisms, and semipurposeful movements do best after surgical resection of the anterior temporal lobe [5]. During the staring spell, the patient clearly has impaired consciousness and does not respond to pain or touch. The stereotyped automatisms include chewing, blinking, swallowing, and similar activities that have repetitious patterns. The semipurposeful movements are coordinated and complex, even if they are inappropriate and performed in a highly reflex manner. These include such banal activities as lighting a cigarette, drinking from a glass, and simple walking around aimlessly [5]. If the seizures originated strictly in the anterior temporal lobe preoperatively, epilepsy may be inapparent in as many as 70 percent of patients 1 year after the surgery, some of them remaining seizure-free on no medication [12]. Up to 50 percent of the individuals who are seizure-free after operation eventually are able to discontinue their use of medication [12].

Those patients who show the least change in or worsening of their epilepsy are those who undergo anterior temporal lobectomy but who exhibit signs of disease outside the temporal lobe. Activities such as conjugate deviation of the eyes to one side early in the ictus or in the aura of the seizure suggest that there is a frontal lobe component to the seizure disorder and are associated with a poor result. If the specimen of brain resected, whether temporal or frontal tissue, reveals no histologic abnormalities, the patient is unlikely to show improvement after the operation [5].

Sectioning of the corpus callosum currently is reserved for patients with poorly defined seizure foci or with seizure foci in highly sensitive areas of the

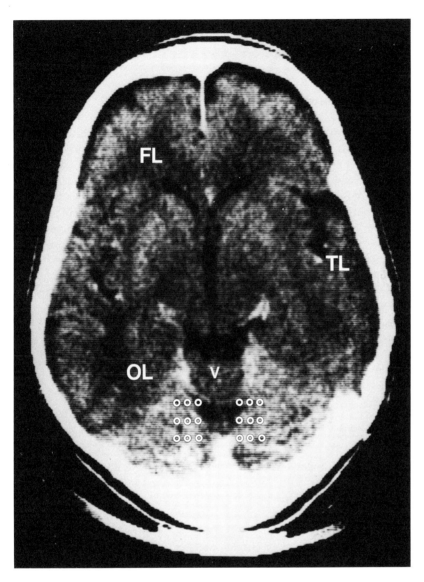

Figure 15–2.
Stimulating electrodes placed over the superior aspect of the lateral hemispheres of the cerebellum (o) have been used with limited success in the management of seizures. The angle of this computed tomogram cuts through the frontal (FL), temporal (TL), and occipital (OL) lobes with inclusion of some posterior fossa structures, such as the vermis (V) and part of the lateral hemispheres of the cerebellum.

brain, such as the principal speech areas. The best results have been seen in patients with childhood-onset generalized seizures. After surgical intervention, these patients still require antiepileptic drugs.

CEREBELLAR STIMULATION

Output from the cerebellum to the thalamus and other structures in the brain is inhibitory, and so it was not surprising that stimulation of the cerebellar cortex in the cat was found to suppress epilepsy [15]. Based upon this observation, several attempts have been made, in patients with intractable seizures, to improve the level of seizure control by implanting electrodes in the posterior cranial fossa overlying the cerebellar cortex (Fig. 15–2) [16]. The surgical procedure used in placing the electrode is minor, and patients seem to tolerate fairly well the foreign objects and the electrical current applied to the electrodes [15]. The results, however, have been inconsistent and largely disappointing.

Patients undergoing cerebellar stimulation may show transient changes in seizure frequency, but there is no pattern to the response, regardless of the stimulus parameters used. An unexpected complication of the procedure is that there is damage to the cerebellar cortex around the area where the electrical stimulus is applied [16]. Cerebellar stimulation is still a strictly experimental approach, and even the few patients who seemed to profit from the technique required antiepileptic medications.

KETOGENIC DIET

A diet designed to make the patient ketotic most of the time has been used for a variety of childhood seizures with some success [17]. It was used in the management of infantile spasms before adrenocorticotropic hormone was introduced, but it has been largely supplanted by this and other drugs for the treatment of infantile spasms. It still is used for some children with intractable minor motor seizures or more common seizure types. It does not appear to be useful in adults, probably because an adult's cerebral metabolism of ketones, such as beta-hydroxybutyrate and acetoacetate, is very different from that in the newborn and infant [17].

A typical ketogenic diet consists of three-fourths fat, one-eighth protein, and one-eighth carbohydrate. Total intake should provide 75 kcal/kg body weight/day, with 1 g of protein per kilogram of body weight figured into the formula [17]. Supplemental vitamins are needed while the child is on this diet. Children started on this diet routinely exhibit hypoglycemia during the first week, but in some children, this hypoglycemia persists and interferes with the child's ability to tolerate the diet [18]. Adjustments must be made in the diet for these children, but little more than an increase in the total calories provided may suffice [18]. Osteomalacia will develop unless the child is given 5,000 IU daily of vitamin D [17]. Alternative diets using medium-chain triglycerides provide more carbohydrates and protein but cause additional gastrointestinal distress [17].

This diet cannot be used in combination with acetazolamide because of the metabolic acidosis that these two agents working together will produce, but most physicians do not use acetazolamide in the management of minor motor seizures [17]. The interaction of valproic acid and the ketogenic diet still is controversial, and so this drug also is best avoided while the child is maintained on the diet. The serum levels of other antiepileptics given to the child while he is on this diet must be closely monitored, as they may increase abruptly after the diet is started [17].

Raising the level of ketones in the blood by eating a diet consisting mostly of vegetable oils and cream will raise the seizure threshold in many children, but the foods allowed are difficult to tolerate even for a few days, and an effective course requires protracted adherence to the diet. The ketogenic diet usually is introduced as a supplement to antiepileptic medication when drugs have failed to suppress seizure activity adequately. It can be continued for months or years if necessary, but most children find it too unpalatable to tolerate.

Many physicians have tried using this diet in adults who have responded poorly to antiepileptic medications, and some claim it has been beneficial. The uncontrolled nature of such observations makes them highly questionable, but the benign character of the diet when used for only a few weeks or months in a young adult may justify its application when the only other real alternative is surgical intervention.

UNCONVENTIONAL TREATMENT

Every individual faced with a life-long burden of medication use or uncertain seizure control hopes for a simple way to eliminate the seizure disorder. This accounts for the appeal of peculiar diets, vitamin regimens, and other folk remedies that range from voodoo ceremonies to hydrotherapy. The eye witness account of a remarkable cure or dramatic improvement in seizure control is more convincing than bland statistics showing that the effect of the megavitamins, holy water, religious conversion, or self-hypnosis did not exceed what would have been expected on the basis of chance alone.

Treatments that are efficacious for some neurologic disorders occasionally are misapplied to the management of epilepsy. Acupuncture has become popular in the management of pain and various addictions, but no amount of enthusiasm can make it effective against epilepsy. Spinal manipulation by a chiropractor also is tried by some patients seeking nonpharmaceutical ways to manage the seizures, but this, too, can have little more than a placebo effect.

Of course, a placebo effect is better than no effect, and so any patient who becomes less disabled with ineffectual, but safe, remedies should not be burdened by his physician's hostility. Whenever the patient insists on using unconventional treatment, the primary physician should advise the patient against approaches that are potentially dangerous and maintain the therapeutic alliance with the patient that will encourage him to continue relying on the physician for advice and treatment.

BIOFEEDBACK

Some success in reducing the number of seizures experienced by patients who have done poorly with antiepileptic medications has been observed with biofeedback [19]. This technique uses operant conditioning to adjust the patient's response to either the seizure aura or to feedback on brain wave activity provided by continuous electroencephalographic recordings [19]. It is safe, except for the risks associated with a patient's discontinuance of his antiepileptic medication use.

Success with the technique varies widely among different centers, and it is clear that the personnel involved in training the patient are as important as the technique itself in determining whether the patient will profit. Currently, it must still be considered of largely theoretical value. The technique is costly and unpredictable, but both of these features may change as more experience is gained in training patients.

TREATMENT OF FACTITIOUS SEIZURES

Factitious seizures do not warrant drug treatment, but most individuals with these seizures are on antiepileptic medications simply because they are thought to have real seizures. Psychiatric intervention is appropriate when the seizures are recognized as factitious. Whatever therapy is instituted must involve both the patient and the people for whom the patient is having seizures. The problem usually cannot be managed if the patient alone is evaluated. Factitious seizures represent a problem with relationships. They generally are more a problem for those obliged to deal with the affected individual than they are for the affected individual himself.

The contrived seizures are meant to secure attention or special consideration, and so they are especially refractory to efforts made to suppress them. Antiepileptic medication usually does not affect the frequency and disruptiveness of the attacks unless the patient is heavily sedated. Confronting the patient with evidence that the seizure activity is not authentic will not stop the behavior but will undermine the relationship betwen the patient and the physician unmasking the factitious complaint. The most effective management involves determining what is prompting the factitious seizures and either eliminating the incentive for the behavior or providing the patient with an alternative behavior that is less disruptive and less dangerous. The special status accorded the victim of the seizure must be eliminated. The attack should be treated as an unfortunate interruption in any activities planned, but it should not be a reason for canceling plans. The patient should be protected from any self-injury during the attack, but the incident should not absolve him or her of any responsibilities [2].

The patient with true seizures who is suspected also of having contrived seizures must be given psychological assistance to minimize the risks of factitious seizures while being continued on the maximally effective anticonvulsant therapy. For patients with strictly factitious seizures, reenacting the seizure scenario is occasionally helpful. The patient is asked to recreate as much as possible the activity typical of a seizure, and the rest of the family behaves as it customarily does during the seizure. Without the excitement and anxiety of a real episode, the role played by each member of the family during an attack becomes more obvious. This may be especially informative when the patient is a child, since interactions between family members are less likely to be disguised or distorted when the seizure victim is a child.

What the individual with contrived seizures actually achieves through the factitious episodes generally is obvious to the physician evaluating them. Techniques to minimize the behavior also are fairly straightforward. Simple devices, such as requiring that every member of the family—not just the one or few desired participants—be present for the entire episode, may change the experience adequately to make it unsatisfying for the individual who contrives the attack. For example, the child who enjoys exclusive access to his or her father at 2:00 a.m. may find little incentive to have nocturnal attacks when each attack brings the entire family to the bedside.

For every patient exhibiting factitious seizures, the primary physician must maintain a level of vigilance that will not allow the patient to suffer an injury even if the seizure is authentic. This vigilance must be accompanied by an evenhanded approach to the patient whenever that person appears sick. The seizure, whether real or contrived, may exempt the patient from responsibilities such as going to work or to school, but it does not entitle him to indulgences. After a real seizure, the patient may be content to do virtually nothing for several hours, but after a contrived seizure, such inactivity may be intolerable. It is unreasonable to allow the child who cannot go to school to sit home and play games or stare at television. To make life with seizures at all rewarding is unwise even when there is little reason to suspect that the seizures are factitious.

Once steps have been taken to make the factitious seizures less rewarding for the patient, the affected individual should be given a respectable and reasonable way out of the so-called seizure problem. A change in drugs or dosages, suggestions that the problem is resolving on its own, and information on biofeedback techniques to modify the sensation preceding a factitious seizure are all strategies available to the primary physician.

GROUP THERAPY

A variety of psychological approaches to the problems fostered by epilepsy are valuable adjuncts to any treatment plan. Most patients do not need individual treatment on a chronic basis, but months of intensive psychotherapy may be required to stabilize the patient in a severe depression [20]. Most people with epilepsy derive great benefit from several different types of group therapy.

The person with epilepsy usually profits from encounters with similarly affected individuals. In groups of people with epilepsy the individual patient at least loses the feeling of isolation that often develops in people with this type of neurologic disorder. The deception and fear of discovery that permeate the life of the individual with marginally controlled epilepsy can be discarded. Discussing problems related to work, family, seizure control, and sexual dysfunction helps defuse them.

Self-deprecation is common when patients with epilepsy enter group discussions with other epileptic individuals, but with continued meetings this usually abates [2]. These patients feel less impaired and generally are less pessimistic when they see how other individuals have handled problems similar to their own. Alliances develop between similarly impaired individuals, and out of these alliances come strategies for dealing with the disorder [2].

The belligerence and animosity that often develop between individuals with epilepsy and their friends and relatives also abate. They continue to resent the fact that they face sanctions, but the smoldering jealousy of people who do not have epilepsy and the self-pity that often develops with chronic disabilities decrease.

When the family of the patient is involved in group meetings with other patients and their families, the strains that develop within the family as a result of the epilepsy can be minimized. The issues most often raised by individuals with epilepsy and their families include adjusting to the illness, relieving tension in the family, planning for the future, balancing dangers faced willingly by the epileptic individual with the desire to feel useful, financial worries, divorce, suicide, changes in social life, living in the present, medication compliance, explaining the illness to other people, alternatives to work, and problems with relatives [2]. Adjusting to the illness means learning to live productively despite the chronic neurologic disorder. For most individuals with poorly controlled seizures, the epilepsy has a paralyzing effect. The constant threat of seizure activity and the increasing, often self-imposed limitation on the individual invariably produce tension in the family. These patients feel that there is no reason to plan for the future, since the epilepsy makes the future seem tenuous.

When boredom or a desire to ignore the chronic problem induces the patient to try routine activities, such as driving, going out alone, or performing routine chores, the family may react by attempting to block this burst of activity [2]. That which seemed harmless and reasonable before the appearance of the epilepsy may now appear dangerous and irresponsible. The conflict that develops between the family members' desire to see the patient become more active and their dread of injury caused by any activity is frequently annoying to the individual with the seizure disorder. Adding to this are the financial worries that seem inescapable when any member of the family has a chronic illness. Some patients consider divorce and even suicide to be legitimate ways of resolving the enormous tension that develops in the family of an epileptic individual.

All these problems require attention, and solutions to them are not feasible in a strictly medical setting. Finding alternatives to a life-style that had to be abandoned because of the seizure disorder is not the responsibility of a physician or a social worker; the alternatives must come from the people who have the problem. If family members participate in group meetings of epileptic patients, a more objective assessment of the actual problems and how they arise is likely to evolve. Clearly, the patient's entire family is affected by the seizure disorder. Enabling these families to meet and explore common dilemmas is more likely to minimize the disruptive effects of the seizures than is monitoring serum antiepileptic levels and adjusting medications.

REFERENCES

1. Delgado-Escueta, A.V., Treiman, D.M., Walsh, G.O. The treatable epilepsies (part 2) *N. Engl. J. Med.* 308(26):1576–1584, 1983.
2. Lechtenberg, R. *Epilepsy and The Family.* Carbridge Mass.: Harvard University Press, 1984.
3. Falconer, M.A., Taylor, D.C. Surgical treatment of drug-resistant epilepsy due to mesial temporal sclerosis. *Arch. Neurol.* 19:353–361, 1968.
4. Van Buren, J.M., Ajmone-Marsan, C., Mutsuga, N., Sadowsky, D. Surgery of temporal lobe epilepsy. *Adv. Neurol.* 8:155–196, 1975.
5. Walsh, G.O., Delgado-Escueta, A.V. Type II complex partial seizures: poor results of anterior temporal lobectomy. *Neurology (N.Y.)* 34(1):1–13, 1984.
6. Falconer, M.A. Reversibility by temporal-lobe resection of the behavioral abnormalities of temporal-lobe epilepsy. *N. Engl. J. Med.* 289:451, 1973.
7. Engel, J., Jr., Driver, M.V., Falconer, M.A. Electrophysiological correlates of pathology and surgical results in temporal lobe epilepsy. *Brain* 98:129–156, 1975.
8. Taylor, D.C. Mental state and temporal lobe epilepsy. *Epilepsia* 13:727–765, 1972.
9. Geschwind, N. Effects of temporal-lobe surgery on behavior. *N. Engl. J. Med.* 289(9):480–481, 1973.
10. Geschwind, N. Aphasia. *N. Engl. J. Med.* 284:654, 1971.

11. Geschwind, N.   Disconnexion syndromes in animals and man. *Brain* 88:237, 585, 1965.
12. Schomer, D.L.   Partial epilepsy. *N. Engl. J. Med.* 309(9):536–539, 1983.
13. Ledoux, J.E., Risse, G.L., Springer, S.P., et al.   Cognition and commissurotomy. *Brain* 100:87–104, 1977.
14. Gazzaniga, M.S.   *The Bisected Brain.* New York: Appleton-Century-Crofts, 1970.
15. Riklan, M., Kabat, C., Cooper, I.S.   Psychological effects of short term cerebellar stimulation in epilepsy. *J. Nerv. Ment. Dis.* 162(4):282–290, 1976.
16. Gilman, S., Bloedel, J., Lechtenberg, R.   *Disorders of the Cerebellum.* Philadelphia: F.A. Davis Co. 1981.
17. DeVivo, D.C.   How to use other drugs (steroids) and the ketogenic diet. In Morselli, P.L., Pippenger, C.E., Penry, J.K. (eds.), *Antiepileptic Drug Therapy in Pediatrics.* New York: Raven Press, 1983, pp. 283–292.
18. DeVivo, D.C., Pagliara, A.S., Prensky, A.L.   Ketotic hypoglycemia and the ketogenic diet. *Neurology* (N.Y.) 23(6):640–649, 1973.
19. Engel, J., Jr., Troupin, A.S., Crandall, P.H. et al.   Recent developments in the diagnosis and therapy of epilepsy. *Ann. Intern. Med.* 97:584–598, 1982.
20. Lechtenberg, R.   *The Psychiatrist's Guide to Diseases of the Nervous System.* New York: John Wiley & Sons, 1982.

Index